The
Informed Health Plan
Act of 2017

A word from author Robert Dennis, MD:

To my fellow concerned citizens,

Thank you for purchasing this book. I am committed to getting this book into the hands of every U.S. legislator and candidate running for national office.

Through my **"Buy One, Send One Free"** campaign, when you purchase a book for yourself, I will send a **free copy** to your legislator or the candidate of your choice.

To send a copy of The Informed Health Plan Act of 2017, please visit:

www.InformedHealthPlan.com

Click on "Send A Free Copy To My Legislator" link in the top right corner.

Add your first name and ZIP Code and we will send a free copy to your legislator.

The Informed Health Plan Act of 2017

A New Healthcare Delivery System for America

Robert Dennis, MD

Published by Robert Dennis ,M.D., P.A.

www.informedhealthplan.com

Cataloging-in-Publication data on file with the Library of Congress

ISBN: 978-0-9974240-1-0
The Informed Health Plan Act of 2017

Printed in the United States of America.

A Word About the Author

Robert Dennis, MD is an orthopaedic surgeon who has practiced medicine for 40 years. He established and developed an orthopaedic surgery practice in Monmouth County, New Jersey, and maintained long-term affiliations with several hospitals in the New York metropolitan area, serving as Director of Orthopaedic Surgery at Jersey Shore University Medical Center, Neptune, NJ.

Dr. Dennis is passionate about his work as a physician, surgeon, inventor, teacher, lecturer and researcher. During the progression of his career, he has witnessed many changes in the field of medicine. Over time, the incremental deterioration of the essence of his profession has been the norm. But in recent years, the intrusion of government has dramatically increased.

The wide sweeping developments in the U.S. healthcare system are what compelled Dr. Dennis to author, in its entirety, The Informed Health Plan Act of 2017. This proposal refutes the assumption that the American consumer is too stupid and incapable of actively participating in their own medical decisions. Dr. Dennis is convinced that the exact opposite is true. This work is a testament to that truth. If adopted, this proposal will harness the individual's proven capabilities to assess value and quality in the deployment of their healthcare dollar just as they do in every other interaction.

This proposal is intended to be politically neutral.

Preface

The Affordable Care Act has
provided some important lessons
on how to implement change,
and now it is time to build on
those lessons.

This proposal defines a solution to the healthcare crisis facing
the United States of America.

Contents

Introduction

Thank you for your interest in this book. The fact that you have purchased **The Informed Health Plan Act of 2017** indicates your concern about the state of the current U.S. healthcare system.

This book explains in detail a new and innovative concept in healthcare delivery. It is my intention to reach the most sincere healthcare legislator, the most sophisticated healthcare expert, the most dedicated physician and most important, the frustrated and bewildered consumer who is paying for it all.

This timely and courageous plan empowers the consumer by offering transparency in pricing, choice in providers, and improvement in quality and a reduction in costs at all levels of health care.

The Informed Health Plan Act accomplishes this by dismantling the bureaucratic machine and shifting these dollars back into the delivery of actual medical care in a simple **two-step** plan:

1. Identify the six stakeholders supporting the current system.

2. Outline the modification of each of their roles in considerable detail.

We have before us a great opportunity to create the world's finest healthcare system. We already have the crucial starting point in place. Simply put, the U.S. already has the most advanced and innovative medicine in the world. What we need to correct is the inefficient, wasteful, inept and exorbitant delivery system. We must make this correction before our country is crushed by the ever-escalating costs of our current healthcare delivery system. We can preserve the good parts of the Affordable Care Act while shedding its excessive bureaucratic burdens.

This effort is dedicated to those who embrace change as the path forward.

Robert Dennis, MD

February 2016

Chapter 1: **Overview**

In order to achieve a health care delivery system that achieves the most desirable goals—defined as *lower costs across the system* and *full access for all*—we must be willing to consider a fundamental restructuring of the American healthcare system.

To expend any effort in this direction and do less at this point would just layer yet another level of complication onto an already over-burdened system in full blown crisis.

The United States' healthcare system is destined for a dramatic change because at the current rate of cost increase it will crush future generations.

This transparent plan empowers consumers to make informed choices and when they do, it captures enormous cost savings.

It is the universal solution, a global approach to a system in crisis.

Outline of key elements

I.   Key Definitions:
  A. Elective care
  B. Urgent care

II. Re-establish fees that reflect actual costs via free market tools

III. Publish fees to establish transparency and enhance marketplace competition

IV. All (rich and poor) have equal access to medical care for all urgent needs

V.   Cost sharing between consumer and insurance companies for elective care needs

VI. Dismantle the bureaucratic machinery, saving trillions of dollars and re-directing that money back into actual medical care

VII. Identify the six integral stakeholders involved in health care delivery and identify the necessary adjustments that each would need to embrace

  A. Government:
    1. Define care as urgent or elective
    2. Establish a web-based free market
    3. Manage means tested insurance for low income
    4. Establish and oversee hospital outreach clinics

B. Insurance companies:
    1. Provide insurance based on only two parameters:
        a. Percent co-pay
        b. Second opinion threshold

C. Hospitals:
    1. Establish and manage outreach clinics
    2. Post and publish all fees for inpatient and outpatient care

D. Providers:
    1. Post and publish current fees and expect free market to adjust

E. Patients/Consumers
    1. Utilize shopping skills to purchase elective medical services
    2. Utilize second opinions in place of third party interference with patient care decisions (substitute confirmatory provider second opinions for micromanagement utilization controls)

F. Attorneys:
    1. Participate in review panel organizations following unsuccessful malpractice litigation to reduce the heavy burden that frivolous suits place on the system

Chapter 2: The Medical Healthcare System Meets the Free Market

What does a test actually cost?

This is the big unknown. Most current pricing evolved from years of layered stealth negotiations between insurers and providers. This has led to artificially inflated prices for patient care visits, testing and procedures.

If we were to re-establish reasonable baseline pricing by allowing providers to price care based on actual costs and permit market competition to continually adjust prices, then we could easily be able to answer that initial question and at the same time unburden the system of tremendous unnecessary bureaucratic costs and artificial inflation.

Only when the consumers of goods and services have access to information that provides for the ability to evaluate cost/benefit and cost/quality calculations, and are spending their own money can the benefit and power of marketplace competition be fully realized. Only then will a free market actually lower costs and improve quality of whatever product or service is being sought.

We challenge the reader to name an industry that creates consumer goods and services where this is untrue.

Why then is this not applicable to medicine?

Rather than explain why it has not applied to the field of medicine in the past, we choose to describe how it should and could apply to all medical services and still preserve the unique aspects of medical care, in particular the existence of life-threatening events (no time to shop), complicated diagnoses that are beyond common or routine, and the need to provide access to medical care for all.

Can a system preserve these unique attributes and still be transparent enough to provide the benefits of the free market system? Namely:

1. Lower cost for everyone

2. Better and more accessible care for everyone

What if such a simple system could be designed to capture the cost-lowering benefits of choice through transparency; the improvement of quality through competition; and at the same time make access to health care even more available to all of society?

Would such a system be worthy of your consideration?

Some successful examples can be cited in other fields where consumers are given meaningful tools and choices.

1. Home Advisors   4. Cars.com

2. Angie's List   5. Carfax

3. Overstock   6. Realtor.com

The list is endless. As an illustration:

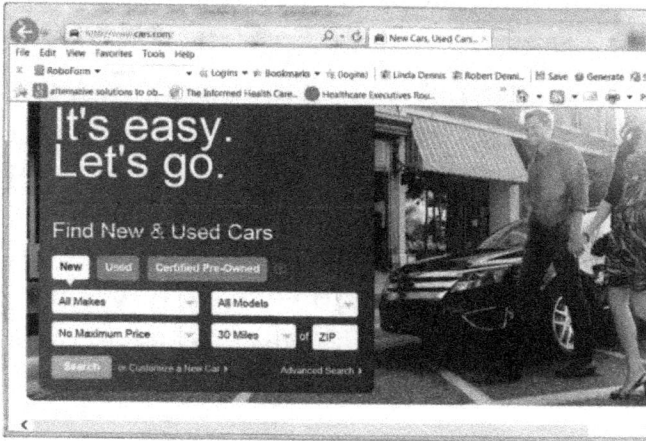

Why not medicine?

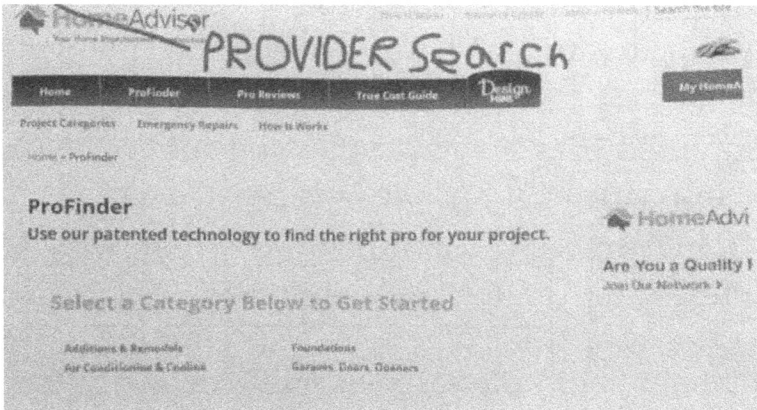

A better question would be:
Why not now in medicine?

The medicine of our fathers is not the medicine of today. Medicine has moved along the same curve of rapid advancement over the past 40 years as has every other industry. Only the structure of the delivery system is stuck in the past; buried in politics, special interests, over-regulation, bureaucracy, lobbyists, outdated legislation, etc.

There are only a few examples where free market competition was allowed to flourish in medicine. For certain types of cosmetic surgery, dental care, pet care, and in the field of eyewear, market competition brought down prices. In fact wherever it has been tried it has always demonstrated the truth of this axiom: **Appropriate competition decreases costs and increases quality.**

So what has changed in these past 40 years that will now allow the bulk of medical care to resemble these other distinct markets?

1. The consumer is smarter and companies already directly market to consumers for complex medical products and medications on TV.
2. Diagnoses have been well-defined and categorized.
3. Specific treatments have been specified for given diagnoses.
4. The Internet is now available and the consumer is well-practiced in making web-based decisions.
5. Various procedures and their indications have been defined and better understood by the consumer and have become more routine (MRI, mammogram, colonoscopy, etc.).
6. Healthcare in general is now part of all of our everyday lives: MRI, colonoscopy, arthroscopy, anti-biotics, total joint replacement, catheterizations and stents are now all common commodities and terms that we all know and understand.

We all enjoy longer and better lives thanks to these advances, but we all also have to agree:

1. The price is too high.
2. The price has not adjusted to the current actual values of different procedures.

In fact, the price has been kept artificially high, much higher than the market would currently value many of these procedures.

Why?

There are two reasons. Both are the result of layered interference by vested interests.

1. The consumer has no reason to shop value versus price.

   He is not spending his own money but rather someone else's; the issue therefore changes from a cost vs. value equation to the feeling that we are all entitled to the best quality of all aspects of medicine at all times with no concern for the cost. This is a simple and predictable result of human nature. (Certainly no big surprise given the way the system is designed.)

2. The system intentionally hides the real prices of the individual goods and services in order to purposely prevent shopping and allows for the designed distortion of prices and access.

To achieve this obscuring of prices, the healthcare system over the past 40 years has developed thousands of new terms, all too familiar to all of us in order to hide, distort, confuse and obscure the cost of what we are actually purchasing. To name just a few:

> Deductibles, provider networks, co-pays, required referrals, EOBs, employer-sponsored programs, ERISA, in-network, out-of-network, denials, delays, maximal medical benefit, IMEs, EMRs, inappropriate procedure, excessive care, penalties, employer mandates, new 3.8% Medicare tax, subsidies, medical necessity, waivers, Cadillac tax, reduced care for end-of-life treatments, IPAB (Independent Payment Advisory Board), Donut Hole, limits of FSA (Flexible Savings Account), ACO (Accountable Care Organization), USPSF (U.S. Preventative Services Task Force).

The list goes on and on.

The more confused the consumer remains and the more docile and passive the consumer can be kept, then the longer the system can perpetuate the interests of the few power stakeholders and their profits.

And who are these stakeholders?

There are only six total stakeholders in all.

Only three are considered power players. Power players are those who most benefit from falsely high costs that are obscured by bureaucracy:

1. **The Insurance Carriers**
2. **The Government**
3. **The Hospital Systems**

Meanwhile, the more important but far less powerful players are of course:

1. **The Patient/Consumer**
2. **The Provider (not just doctors)**
3. **The Attorneys (behind the scenes but nonetheless cost drivers)**

What's wrong with this picture?

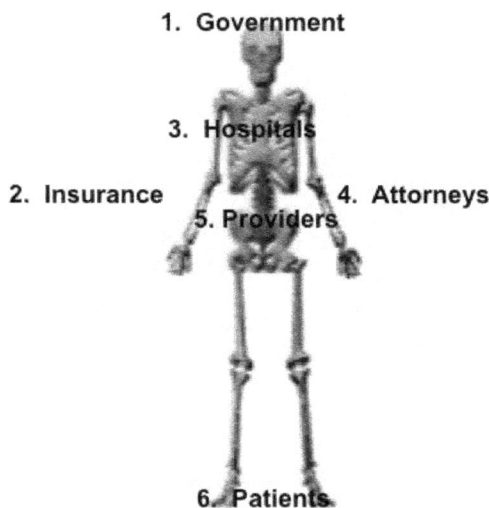

1. Government
2. Insurance
3. Hospitals
4. Attorneys
5. Providers
6. Patients

The patient should be at the top, not the government!

Robert Dennis, MD

Chapter 3: "Just Imagine"

"All the things we achieve are things we have first of all imagined."

David Malouf (Australian writer)

There are always new opportunities to correct mistakes and to do better. But as we have learned from the Affordable Care Act, the devil is in the details and we have to really understand something and own it before we should implement it. This plan promises to comply with the first group of items on the list below, in order to achieve the desired outcomes in the second list.

Devil in the Details
It's not what we see, but what we don't see

1. No referrals
2. No provider networks
3. No authorizations
4. No re-pricing
5. No denials
6. No post service denials
7. No delays in payment

We all want:
1. Lower costs
2. Access for all people
3. Fair reimbursement
4. Less bureaucracy
5. Less unnecessary litigation
6. Any licensed provider
7. Decrease <u>unnecessary</u> care and waste
8. Minimize complications
9. One Fee

This proposal explains exactly how we can achieve these goals. It will challenge even the most adventurous among us to rethink the entire system.

Chapter 4: Today vs. Tomorrow: A Typical Consumer Interaction

What if your doctor suggests you should get a colonoscopy?

In today's system you look in your plan and go to the provider your insurance plan directs you to, who is in your network. You then call to make an appointment and confirm that they accept your insurance.

The provider may be far from your home, but you have little to say about their location or qualifications. You have no other choices. In other words, you go where you are told, knowing little of the quality and nothing of the costs or the charges that a particular provider may bill your insurance company. You know even less about what they're likely to pay him or her. If your co-pay is a percentage of the provider's fee, you would have no idea what that means in actual dollars since his fee is invisible to you. You do not know what the facility charge will be or what the anesthesiologist might charge. More importantly, you would only be hoping that the anesthesiologist is in your network.

In other words, as a consumer this becomes a totally blind item, as you are only responsible for the co-pay plus some unknown additional amount. At this point you have no idea of what that co-pay amount might be. You're not sure of anything, but then again they don't expect you to care about the cost, after all... it's not your money! Or is it?

Despite the fact that you now know all about the procedure

because you looked it up on the Internet, you remain totally in the dark as to whether or not you really need a colonoscopy at this moment in time and how much it is really going to cost you, or your insurance company, and the effect it may have on your future premiums. And for that matter, you're not even sure who will learn of the results or how they will be disseminated through the electronic medical records and how this might be detrimental to your future access to healthcare coverage, employment, life insurance policy purchases, license applications, etc.

Now just imagine that your insurance plan was transparent for this elective procedure and your co-pay, let's say, was 10% of the actual cost of this service. (This was the co-pay percentage you chose when you bought the insurance.)

(As we will explain later on, in this new plan the consumer selects the co-pay percentage with which he is comfortable when he chooses his insurance plan.)

The website from which you purchased insurance might have looked like this:

User Friendly Window: Consumer Insurance
How Do Patients Select Insurance?

Percent Co-pay (PC)	Second Opinion Threshold (SOT)	ZIP Code	Compare Price
Consumer Selects	Consumer Selects		
15% (PC)	$1,000 (SOT)	07757	$300/month IC 1 $200/month IC 2 $150/month IC 3 xxxx - IC 4 - Not available in that price range

The website from which you could have access to shop the provider and procedure might look like this:

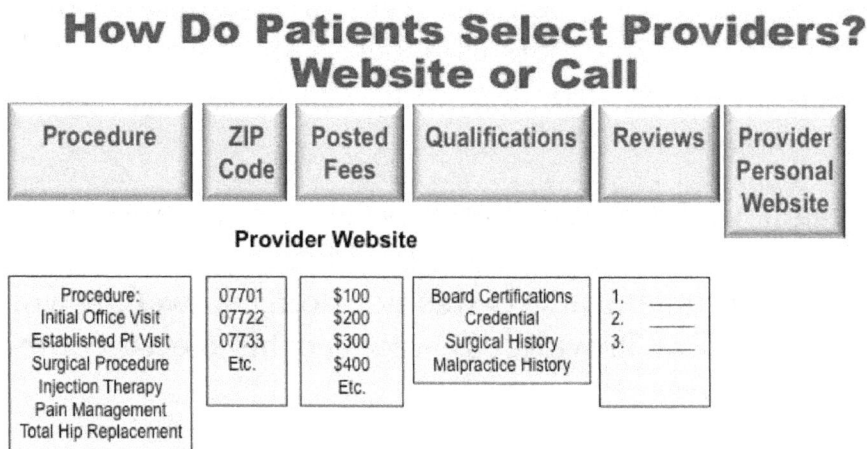

How Do Patients Select Providers? Website or Call

Procedure	ZIP Code	Posted Fees	Qualifications	Reviews	Provider Personal Website

Provider Website

Procedure: Initial Office Visit Established Pt Visit Surgical Procedure Injection Therapy Pain Management Total Hip Replacement	07701 07722 07733 Etc.	$100 $200 $300 $400 Etc.	Board Certifications Credential Surgical History Malpractice History	1. ____ 2. ____ 3. ____

Free market will define fees and winners and losers
Providers can change fees annually

Now assume the Informed Health Plan Act (IHPA of 2017) has become law.

Your doctor suggests you should get a colonoscopy.

You are a modern patient/consumer. You go to the single government-sponsored website that provides the listings of all the providers in your area that perform colonoscopies, their credentials, their patient feedback stars as well as the fees that each of those providers and facilities and preferred anesthesiologists will accept.

These fees have nothing to do with your particular insurance plan (there are no networks). These fees would be the same if you paid cash, had Obamacare, or any other insurance plan.

These fees would be the same if you had no insurance or were underinsured. These single fees would be the same if you had a green card, a blue card, or no card.

These same fees are visible to not only all consumers but also to the provider's competitors who, over a short period of time, would quickly adjust their fees to accommodate competition vs. volume issues.

If a colleague was attracting patients, and the patient schedule of Provider "A" was full, while Provider "B" with the same credentials and qualifications was not doing so well, it would not be long before Provider "B" reduced his fee to compete effectively.

As we will explain later on, in this new plan the consumer searches the procedure website for the desired procedure, identifies his ZIP Code, and searches for a provider of his choice based on quality and price. (Both the provider search and the procedure search website would be similar.) This would only take a few clicks. All willing licensed providers would be listed.

There are no networks, no referrals needed, no artificial state line restrictions, no third party in the room between you and your provider and nothing prohibiting you from moving forward or not.

The first page of the website might look something like this:

How Do Patients Select Providers?
Website or Call

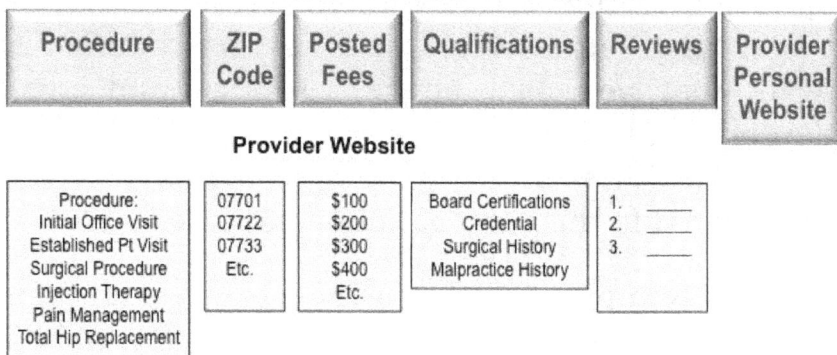

Procedure	ZIP Code	Posted Fees	Qualifications	Reviews	Provider Personal Website

Provider Website

Procedure: Initial Office Visit Established Pt Visit Surgical Procedure Injection Therapy Pain Management Total Hip Replacement	07701 07722 07733 Etc.	$100 $200 $300 $400 Etc.	Board Certifications Credential Surgical History Malpractice History	1. ____ 2. ____ 3. ____

Free market will define fees and winners and losers
Providers can change fees annually

Three clicks later, you select the provider of your choice at the price you wish to pay and make an appointment.

Some may want the cheapest, some consumers may want the most expensive, some consumers may want the best by credentials and feedback, and some consumers may not care or just want the closest.

It's your choice!

But the best part is yet to come. Let's dissect this single issue of elective care just a little further and understand the impact it will have on the cost of care for the whole system.

Because this new transparent healthcare delivery system was available, and within three clicks, your shopping effort and skill has not only saved you serious money but it has also dramatically affected the cost of that colonoscopy to your insurer, who has to pay the other 90% of the fees. You certainly worked no harder than you would have to get the best price and quality of a TV, refrigerator, or an airline ticket, so why not use the same intuitive and intelligent purchasing skills to purchase an elective medical procedure? The difference is that you had access to price and quality information related to a TV or a refrigerator, and because of the Informed Health Plan Act (IHPA) you had that same information related to the purchase of health care.

Let's take the example a little further so we can better understand the massive impact this simple system could have on lowering medical costs across the board.

The key is that your co-pay was a percentage of the provider's posted fee. At the annual renewal of your health care insurance policy, your healthcare insurance provider (also part of this new transparent system) offered you co-pays, as did their competitors, that ranged from 3% to 30% of the providers' posted fee.

We assumed for the purpose of this example that you chose a 10% co-pay. The website listed several providers of colonoscopy.

1. Dr. A's posted fee was $2000, the facility where he works posted a fee of $6000, and the anesthesiologist that he works with posted a fee of $1000. To choose Dr. A meant that you would have a colonoscopy for a total cost of $9,000.

   The cost to you would be $900; this would give you the procedure performed by the doctor of your choice.

2. Dr. B's posted fee was $5000, the facility where he works

Robert Dennis, MD

posted a $10,000 fee, and the anesthesiologist (you could have chosen separately) charged $3000, for a total cost of $18,000 (double).

The cost to you if you had chosen Dr. B would therefore be $1800.

You saved $900 (that's real money in your pocket) in this transparent system by using your shopping skills for this elective procedure.

But the best part is that you were able to provide a dramatic systemwide total cost reduction via your shopping abilities. The insurance company that sold you the policy is obligated to pay the other 90% of the provider's posted fee. You just saved your insurance company $9000. This multiplied 1000s of times across the board for elective procedures gives you a glimpse of the real power and benefit of transparent competition and consumer choice. Even better is the fact that the insurance carrier had little if any bureaucratic overhead costs in this process nor did the provider. The system saved a huge amount of bureaucratic overlay. Best of all, you suffered no delays or denials.

You provided the system a huge savings and the system provided you the ability to save significantly in your medical care, while allowing you to choose your provider. It's that simple!

Multiply this 1 million times. Even if it doesn't work for everyone, it will certainly work for cost-conscious consumers.

The power of your shopping capabilities saved the entire system both bureaucratic and overhead costs as well as actual costs. The providers received the fee that they were willing to accept with minimal hassle. The provider and insurance carrier were freed of tremendous bureaucratic overhead and benefited from dramatically lower cost. In fact, all parties involved experience a benefit. (Currently the bureaucratic costs to deliver medical care range from 25 to 45% of the medical dollar, so these savings are no small part of getting you much more value and a much larger percentage of medical care for your medical dollar.)

Eventually all parties will benefit from the competitive marketplace by the effect that all players have on adjusting fees to realistic figures. **This portion of the envisioned healthcare program is exclusively reserved for elective care only.** Please keep in mind that the vast majority of medical costs are spent on the elective side of the ledger.

Chapter 5: The Second Opinion for Elective Care: Better utilization control

Now let's look at the other side of this equation. As an informed consumer wouldn't you also want to ask your provider who suggested the colonoscopy why you needed it and why you need it now?

Perhaps you had reason to question if it could be postponed. For example, maybe you only had one five months ago and it was negative as far as you were told. A second opinion will give you more comfort than a bureaucrat in some insurance building looking at an algorithm, plugging in your age, and then sending you a denial letter.

In this system, a second opinion is always your option, is encouraged, and in some cases, even required. For example, if you had purchased insurance with a second opinion threshold of $10,000, and you were considering a very expensive procedure such as total hip replacement, a confirmatory second opinion can be required for an elective procedure.

A second opinion, by a doctor of your own choosing with qualifications at your comfort level, is a critical part of this system. The fee you might pay for the second opinion would be trivial in the scope of things and in comparison to the fees you would pay for a perhaps unnecessary colonoscopy or a premature total hip replacement. A second opinion is always a good thing, and in this new system, functions as a substitute for all the redundant algorithms and layered bureaucratic medicine that we all deal with currently.

For a second opinion you would select the doctor from the same website. The website would display all the physician's consultation fees. You would simply select the physician whose consultation fee was within your budget. Yes, of course, you have to pay the same 10% when you go for that second opinion. A second confirmatory consultation may cost perhaps $200. Your 10% co-pay would expose you to $20.

You benefit with a meaningful valid second opinion which replaces piles of paperwork and unnecessary bureaucracy and personnel. This second opinion can only accrue to your benefit. If you like the second doctor, there is no prohibition, within this system, that would prevent you from staying with the second doctor, based on your comfort level.

If the second doctor agrees with the first doctor, and you decide to proceed with the procedure, the system may reward you by refunding all or a portion of the percent co-pay you expended when you proceeded with the final procedure.

On the other hand, if the second opinion doctor disagreed and felt that you did not need that procedure, but you chose to go ahead with it anyway, that is also okay; it will always be your choice. The second opinion physician is not there to prevent you from getting an appropriate procedure, but to offer an alternative opinion as a method to help prevent you from proceeding with an unnecessary procedure.

This method of utilization review is better than any alternative algorithm or committee decision as is the case with the Affordable Care Act and its Independent Payment Advisory Board (IPAB), an elected board empowered to reduce what hospitals and doctors are paid, created within the Obama Administration.

Robert Dennis, MD

The doctor who said you need a colonoscopy or total hip procedure will know (because he also participates in the system) that you are going for a second opinion, because you have to, and therefore he may try harder to accommodate you, improve his bedside manner or shorten his wait times, even though his posted fee will continue to compete with those of his colleagues.

It will be your choice totally. This cannot hurt and is far better than the current bureaucratic method of questioning the medical necessity of every recommended elective procedure. That second consultation may save you money, time and perhaps even save you an unnecessary procedure. The second doctor may offer you an alternative option or a less dramatic pathway to wellness. This can only be a good thing for you. Most would think that the $20 would be money well spent.

Definitions & Abbreviations
What is meant by SOT?

Second Opinion Threshold = SOT:

The cost of care (as posted) over which a patient agrees to simply consult with another prescribing provider (of his choice and of the same specialty) to discuss his options in regards to a considered elective procedure, test, device, or drug.

Yes, the patient will have to pay his percent co-pay to the 2nd opinion provider (after having considered that provider's posted fee). **He gets a real 2nd opinion and the original procedures, if he so wishes**, for the price of the % co-pay.

What is missing from this entire system is deductibles, referrals, authorizations, delays and millions if not billions of dollars of administrative costs and frustration.

Chapter 6: Affordable Care for All Life- and Limb-Threatening Conditions

The Affordable Care Act (ACA) was the first experiment in trying to take advantage of the incredible medical progress made over the past 40 years. It served a very good purpose. It demonstrated that a major change can be implemented and is possible. If the next major change that is made in the system achieves the promises made by the Affordable Care Act, then there is still hope for a better healthcare delivery system. American consumers might yet even yearn for, be receptive to, and willing to try another experiment, particularly if the characteristics of the plan were understood, transparent and just plain simpler. The Affordable Care Act did demonstrate the value of the Internet and its application to modern medicine.

So what is the best alternative?

A balanced mix of free market transparent choice for elective procedures and a slightly more traditional approach with government oversight and participation in the cost of care for life-threatening situations. To be sure, these two separate parts of medical care need to be kept separate, thought of as separate and unique, and be clearly differentiated!

Even the phrase "healthcare system for all" is not the same as "health care for all."

What do we mean? You can't force people into health and penalize them or their physicians if they do not do exactly what you want. You can make health care available for everyone and provide an equal playing field for all citizens/consumers.

This new imaginative form of a healthcare delivery system can not only be a great cost reducer but can also achieve all the goals of society in this modern era.

On the other hand, "health care for all" will guarantee marked cost increases across the board and lower both the quality of and the access to medical care for everyone.

A "healthcare system for all" will do the exact opposite and achieve the required and desired goals. So let's be clear and careful about what we ask for because we might get it.

This new system could be put in the form of an act similar to the Affordable Care Act. It can be implemented alongside of the Affordable Care Act as another choice or an eventual replacement for the Affordable Care Act. Given the choice, we believe the majority of consumers will choose this new imaginative option. For the purposes of this publication we will call this the **Informed Health Plan Act of 2017** (IHPA of 2017).

It can be fully described well within perhaps no more than 300 pages as opposed to the 3000 pages of the Affordable Care Act. The 300 pages in simple language would replace the incomprehensible, legalese babble embedded in the Affordable Care Act.

This proposed Informed Health Plan Act of 2017 with the help of actuaries can be quantitatively tagged and easily demonstrate enormous cost savings. It would build on the technology, diagnosis codes and procedure codes that are already well-established. It would make full use of the fraud detection systems that are already solidly in place and wouldn't require penalties. It would be easy to roll out and not require thousands upon thousands of confusing pages to understand. Most importantly, it would never leave the details up to unelected stealthy bureaucrats to manipulate by allowing them to fabricate the rules and regulations. The free market will do that.

For the purpose of overview we will list the key characteristics and benefits of this imaginative new healthcare delivery system.

Key Characteristics of
The Informed Health Plan

✓ Alternative Healthcare Delivery System and Revolutionary Comprehensive Concept

✓ Covers EVERYONE – rich and poor

✓ Free-market driven

✓ Dramatically lowers healthcare costs

✓ Achieves ALL that Affordable Care intended

✓ New concept revolves around DEFINITIONS of elective care vs. urgent and catastrophic care (rather then mandates and penalties)

✓ Easy to understand and implement

✓ Enhances patient's choice and the doctor/patient relationship

✓ Assumes that both rich and poor are equally able to make informed healthcare decisions (in the same way that we decide which TV, food, or appliance to purchase) – value vs. price (we are good at this)

✓ Relies on legitimate second opinions instead of rationing committees, government penalties, subsidies, referrals, authorizations, provider networks, deductibles and bureaucratic obstructions, etc.

Robert Dennis, MD

Chapter 7: The System's Linchpin: The Critical Line Between Urgent Care and Elective Care

The critical line that makes this system work is a line that is already well-established and easily understood in medicine and can be quickly formalized and detailed.

It is the line between acute care and elective care.

The definition of acute care is simply any care that addresses any life-threatening or limb-threatening issue.

Examples of life or limb-threatening care:

- Catastrophic care
- Cancer care
- Acute cardiac care including cardiac catheterization, stents and angioplasties
- Acute pulmonary care
- Fracture care

Anything that threatens life or limb either in the short-term or long-term, including a situation/condition in which delayed treatment might jeopardize life or limb.

The exact, well laid-out and fully described definition of such care will be left to specialty experts and government panels, and will be modifiable from time to time and published for all to see by a Government Panel set up within the Informed Health Plan Act of 2017 (IHPA). There will be a built-in place for meaningful feedback and recommendations that will allow for improvement over time.

The definition of elective care is very simple: all other care that is not defined above. (Most money is spent on the elective care portion of medical costs.)

Examples of elective care:

- Any care that can wait or is non-urgent
- Any routine testing or exams
- Long-term management of illnesses such as diabetes or arthritis
- Anything that can wait without incurring dire consequences (anything where there is sufficient time for a second opinion; a condition that might have gone on for any length of time and where allowing it to go on for some additional time will not be detrimental to the patient)
- Such procedures as MRIs, CT scans
- Arthroscopies
- Total hip replacements
- Total knee replacements
- Pain management
- Most psychiatric issues, etc.

Robert Dennis, MD

How is the <u>Definition of Elective Care</u> & Urgent/Catastrophic Decided?

Urgent & Catastrophic Care:	Elective Care:
All care that is life-saving or limb-saving	All care that is <u>NOT</u> life-threatening or limb-threatening

✓ Each specialty lists which diagnosis and which procedures (using current codes) are life-saving and limb-saving in their specialty

✓ HHS approves the lists and publishes the list on the web and in hard copy to all providers and public (revisable every 2 years)

Chapter 8: Definitions and abbreviations made simple

To assist in the understanding of some specific terms that will be repeated in this overview, please take a close look at the following:

Summary of Abbreviations
To be used in this concept

P   = Provider

PF = Posted Fee

PC = % Co-pay

SOT = Second Opinion Threshold

EC = Elective Care

UC = Urgent & Catastrophic Care

UC = Urgent Care or catastrophic care or emergency care has already been well defined as life-threatening, limb-threatening life-limiting.

EC = Elective Care has already been well described in previous chapters.

P = Provider refers to any and all medical providers, not just physicians but also nurses, hospitals, chiropractors, EMTs, clinics and surgery centers, etc.

Definitions & Abbreviations

Posted Fees = PF

Those fees required to be posted by **every** provider for **all** the goods and services they provide on **all** published schedules in the order of frequency provided. Providers set their own fees and will **compete** in the marketplace for price with other providers of the same service in their same **zip code**. (They can change their fees annually based on supply and demand.)

% Copay = PC:

The percent of the posted fee that the patient has selected (when he chooses his insurance) that he agrees to pay to the provider.

OR

The percent copay that was assigned to him/her by a uniform means test at the hospital outreach clinic.

Robert Dennis, MD

Definitions & Abbreviations
What is meant by SOT?

Second Opinion Threshold = SOT:

The cost of care (as posted) over which a patient agrees to simply consult with another prescribing provider (of his choice and of the same specialty) to discuss his options in regards to a considered elective procedure, test, device, or drug.

Yes, the patient will have to pay his percent co-pay to the 2nd opinion provider (after having considered that provider's posted fee). **He gets a real 2nd opinion and the original procedures, if he so wishes**, for the price of the % co-pay.

What is missing from this entire system is deductibles, referrals, authorizations, delays and millions if not billions of dollars of administrative costs and frustration.

Understanding these simple new terms represents all that will be required in order to understand the entire concept.

Please refer to these pages as we go into more detail, utilizing these abbreviations to easily and visually explain the actuarial assumptions that provide for the funding and full explanation of an implementation of this plan.

Chapter 9: The Special Role of Government

The role of government will be several-fold, as follows:

1. **To create** and continually update the definitions of life- threatening or limb-threatening listed procedures utilizing well-established diagnoses and procedure codes.

2. **To define** and continually update a nationally published, per state, means test to be applied to uninsured and underinsured residents. A simple actuarial derived graph of income versus percent co-pay and confirmatory second opinion threshold that hospital intake centers would apply uniformly to individual patients applying for assisted or government coverage. This will be explained in more detail in later chapters.

3. **Establish and oversee the outreach clinics** required to be established by each hospital to care for the underinsured and uninsured patients that have acquired an assisted or government coverage insurance card.

4. **Establish and maintain fraud and abuse guidelines** in appropriate places within the system, many of which have already been well-identified.

5. **Establish and maintain national informational**

public websites with secure provider portals. Through one website, providers can list the fees that they will accept for all the procedures that they do in the order of frequency. A second website provides complete information on the credentials, qualifications, licenses, procedure histories, malpractice history and patient feedback ratings of each provider. These websites are to be available to all.

Given that the government is already experienced with the intricacies of setting up a website and have by now learned the process well, one might anticipate that these challenges would not be overwhelming.

How Does Assigned Insurance Work?

Go to Hospital &/or Hospital Outreach Clinic Intake/Reception

Sum of All Sources of Income $____ $____ $____ Total $__	Proof of Income _____ _____ _____ _____	Zip _____	Sign Fraud Statement "I affirm under penalty of the law..." Yes ____ No ____	Means PC _____ _____ _____ _____	Means SOT _____ _____ _____ _____

Who Can Apply for Assigned Insurance?
Anyone or Everyone

Means tested income will likely produce higher PC & SOT than private carriers for wealthier patients

Chapter 10: The Six Stakeholders

It is important to acknowledge that healthcare delivery is substantially affected by six unique participants, all of whom have reason to want to protect their own interest or turf. However, any serious effort to reform health care has to identify and to some extent modify the manner in which all six of these participants impact the system.

There is a reason that we dedicated this book to those who embrace change as the path forward. Change is the hardest request we can make of any individual.

Any change in the system must incorporate and require change in the way all six participants provide and receive benefit. We have previously identified the six players and separated the three power players from the non-power players in the roles that they currently hold. Understand that none of the players who have already staked out positions in the current system will invite a change that will alter roles that they had so ardently fought for. But change must come because the system has collapsed before our eyes, no longer providing health care in the way we need to receive it. Future generations should not be asked to pay for our unwillingness to act.

The Informed Health Plan Act represents a sea change in the manner that healthcare delivery will be carried out. Therefore, one must anticipate full-fledged resistance in the form of detailed criticism of every aspect of this reform. However, for the better good it is hoped that all six players will be able to look beyond their specific prejudices and appreciate that they are being asked to change on an equal basis. Some will acknowledge beneficial change as it applies to the other five, and some will scream that the changes that apply to them are negative. However, if all six players are willing to think out-of-the-box, then the system will benefit everyone, and their own benefits will ultimately far surpass the changes they are being asked to consider individually.

We will describe these changes in the form of new rules for each stakeholder.

We previously discussed the role that the government would play in this new system. Next, we will examine all six players and describe the role modification required for each one. When taken together, a dramatic new system will emerge from the current shattered and dysfunctional system.

The players in order of importance are:

1. The Patient

2. The Provider

3. The Hospitals

4. The Insurance Carriers

5. The Government

6. The Attorneys

Let's review this diagram again that is labeled with the six players:

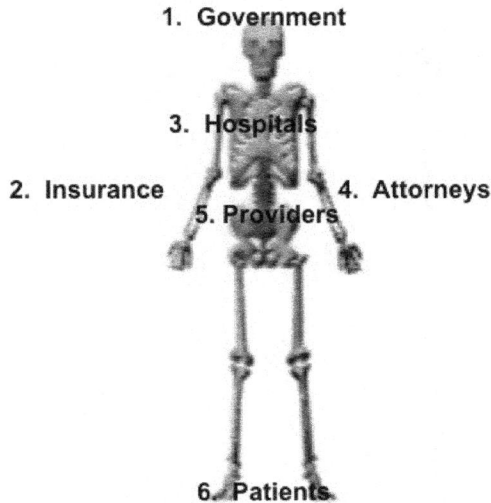

What's wrong with this picture?

1. Government
3. Hospitals
2. Insurance
4. Attorneys
5. Providers
6. Patients

ALL SIX PLAYERS WILL BE AFFECTED BY CHANGE

1. New Rules
2. Advantages
3. Disadvantages
4. Medicare to be untouched for 10 years

However, purely for the purposes of better understanding of the system, we will present the changes that each player must make in the order that the reader can best understand the whole picture.

New Rules and Details

1. Government
2. Insurance Companies
3. Hospitals
4. Attorneys
5. Providers
6. Patients

GOVERNMENT: New Rules

1. Clearly provide the definitions of urgent, catastrophic and elective care

2. Fund in large measure two distinct pools of money (that any provider or hospital can access if the care provided meets the definitions): **Urgent and/or Catastrophic Pool** and **Uninsured Pool**

3. Define a Means Test

4. Set up and manage two large comprehensive websites: **Provider Fees and Provider Qualifications**

Details: Government

A. Fully and clearly define **terms** (for all to know and abide by)

    1. Catastrophic, urgent (life-saving or limb-saving care), which combined presently represent the smaller portion of medical costs.

    2. Non-urgent care, which is **ALL** care not defined as **urgent** or **catastrophic**. (This currently represents the majority of medical costs.)

    3. **All care** determined to be catastrophic care is to be paid for by the catastrophic care pool for all patients whether they have insurance or not (without having

to pay any co-pay). The fund will pay 100% of such care.

4. The means test that clinics and hospitals use to delineate what amount uninsured patients who appear for care at hospital outreach clinics will have to pay, if anything.

5. Define "practical frivolous lawsuits" exclusively for medical malpractice cases (see **Attorneys**). (Litigation that failed and that has been found to be frivolous by both medical and legal peer review panels as will be described in a later chapter.)

B. **LEAVE MEDICARE ALONE:** Tax whoever you have to, but do it transparently and identify the source of revenues.

C. Investigate and prosecute cases of suspected fraud, system abuse, or over-treatment especially as related to medical/legal cases and other types of criminal behavior that constitute stealing from the system. (Laws are already in place but not vigorously enforced.)

D. Design and manage two important websites that will include **ALL** providers of medical care. **One for fees and one for qualifications**; both sorted by any of several variables.

E. Lift prohibition against suing HMO's.

F. Fund, in combination with state government, hospital-run outreach clinics through an "**Uninsured Care Pool.**"

This pool will be funded by a combination of contributions from:

- Federal Government
- State Government
- Private Insurance companies
- Philanthropic Organizations
- Patients who access these hospital outreach clinics according to a uniformly applied "means test"

G. Fund, in combination with insurance carriers and state governments, a pool titled **"Catastrophic Care Pool."**

H. The government must clearly identify the revenue sources and taxes being levied to support this "Uninsured Care Pool" as well as the "Catastrophic Care Pool."

I. Expand and devise health saving plans for employees **and individuals.**

J. Extend COBRA and provide tax credit for individuals who purchase healthcare insurance to the same extent as groups of employees enjoy when they purchase health care through their employers. (This biased government tax supplement should be removed so the playing field can be equalized and blind to where the insurance was purchased.)

K. Enact tort reform as described in the section titled "Attorneys."

L. Direct and regulate hospitals and patients to abide by definitions of catastrophic and urgent care. Require hospital emergency rooms to direct all care determined to be **"non-urgent care" to their outreach clinics or to the patients' private doctors.**

This will allow hospital Emergency Rooms to take care of only urgent and catastrophic care and redirect all other care. This will save millions and yet provide appropriate care to both the uninsured and the insured.

1. If the patient presents to the Emergency Room and needs urgent care, the Emergency Room provides it and bills the Urgent Care Fund their full fee (no co-pays are billed to the patient).

   a. If the patient is admitted, the hospital bills the Urgent Care Fund in the same manner. The patient will not be responsible for any part of such care.

   b. If it turns out that the care was not for urgent issues, then the bills are directed to the private insurer or Uninsured Fund and the patient will be responsible for the appropriate co-pay accordingly (large hospital bills, as addressed later, are appropriately reduced.)

   c. The Government monitors and polices this process just as they do now.

2. If the patient presents to the Emergency Room and requires non-urgent care, the Emergency Room is not to initiate care, but rather redirect that patient (whether insured or not) to:

   a. Their outreach clinic at which time a means test will be applied, if they are uninsured.

b. Their private provider if they are insured. where they will pay the co-pay that they selected when they signed up for their insurance.

M. Eliminate pre-authorization/precertification and referrals, along with all the bureaucracy and costs associated.

N. (Optional) Regulate subrogation mechanism to expedite a true one payer system to incorporate:

1. Worker's compensation indemnity

2. Auto Insurance

3. Federally mandated programs, etc. (So that there is only one payer and mechanism for health care for all people regardless of when or how they were injured or how they contracted a certain illness.)

O. Regulate healthcare insurers to conform to these new rules.

INSURANCE COMPANIES:
New Rules

1. Eliminate the huge internal bureaucracies by paying for second opinions, both voluntary and mandatory, as utilization review. This would include eliminating items such as referrals, authorizations, deductibles, denials, and provider networks)

2. Establish competitive premiums on the basis of only two parameters:

    a. The amount of co-pay the patient chooses

    b. The threshold level that triggers a mandatory specialty-specific second opinion

Details: Insurance Companies

A. Provide catastrophic insurance separately delineated as a specific portion of the premium charged and provide such catastrophic funds to National Catastrophic Pool. Based on some proportion to be shared with the government and other voluntary supporters, this pool will pay for all catastrophic care.

B. Pay 100% of all care of their insureds that fits the government definition of urgent care with no co-pay or no second opinions necessary via its contribution to the Urgent Care Fund, seen as a line item on each insured's annual premium invoice.

Provide a portion of their premium (line item, clear and transparent) for uninsured care to go to a pool along with government funds to support hospital outreach clinics to cover their share of medical care for the poor. This pool will receive insurance company funds as well as government funds and patient payments (based on a uniform means test) as well as charitable contributions.

C. Provide insurance for non-urgent care (the majority of medical care is non-urgent) with 1% to 30% co-pay (depending on the specific policy). Co-pays are to be paid on all bills where elective care is provided. (No care can be completely free if a patient has insurance. We all must have "skin in the game.") Even if the co-pay is very small, it must be applied to all bills.

Whatever the co-pay that the patient selects, the hospital charges for all elective care. However, as will be described later, hospital co-pay percentages will be dramatically further discounted to avoid excessive patient burdens.

As people attempt to decrease their small portion of their own bills (and now have the tools to do so), they will automatically decrease the insurance company's larger portion of the bills. The fees will drop substantially within the first several years of the institution of this new law as a function of the free market.

Insurance companies will therefore have to sell policies on the basis of only two criteria:

1. % of co-pay the patient chooses for elective care;
2. Threshold amount for non-urgent services that require a second opinion (see Section IV under 'Patient')

All other issues that obstruct care will disappear (networks, providers, deductibles, provider negotiated fees, mandatory IMEs, need for referrals, need for authorization, etc.). Finally, patients will be able to compare and shop insurance.

D. Deductibles will be eliminated. No more deductibles. (Deductibles serve to only cloud issues and prevent patients from understanding true costs.)

E. Must sell Medical Savings Insurance Plans substantially lower than HMO or PPO types of plans. (In other words, provide incentives to encourage people to purchase.) Savings plan insurance is critical, and some forms are already in place. The laws governing such plans are not to be changed.

F. No exclusions for pre-existing conditions (no more cherry picking).

G. No differential between group or individual plans (no more games).

H. All plans must be portable state-to-state and regulated at the federal level (like many other industries). This means that any state licensed provider can see any patient (as it should be).

1. At first, contracted and subcontracted networks must be cross-credentialed or related

in such a way as to be seamless to the patients, state-to-state. (No more networks or at first invisible networks.)

2. Therefore, the patient, the system and the free market will replace the insurance companies/providers' closed-door negotiations (transparency and free market will be allowed to work properly).

I. **Extend COBRA** substantially.

J. **Simplify** plans so that they can be understood by all patients. (EOBs should have two columns, what you paid and what they paid.)

This plan will eliminate pre-authorization/pre-certification and referrals, along with all the bureaucracy and associated costs.

K. Track, identify and provide information for investigation and prosecution of the appropriate agencies when patterns of behavior that suggest medical/legal insurance fraud (doctor, patient, carrier, or attorney) are detected.

L. (Optional) A single healthcare payer for all health care (other than Medicare), no fault (auto insurance) and worker's compensation requiring carriers to reciprocate and subrogate behind the scenes among each other (so no other laws will need to be changed) all at the same posted fees. Separate indemnity payments from medical care. All the same rules apply for indemnity payments. Handle through carrier-to-carrier transactions behind the scenes.

- A precipitous drop in car insurance costs and in

workers' compensation premiums will be realized immediately and will be a huge boost to the economy.

- Employer's premiums for workers' compensation insurance will drop.
- All purchasers of auto insurance will enjoy large and immediate savings.
- Hundreds of millions of dollars will be saved.

Summary: Insurance companies will compete on two key parameters:

1. Premiums associated with a given co-pay, 1% to 30%. The higher the co-pay, the smaller the premium.

2. Premiums associated with a patient-selected second opinion threshold. The smaller the threshold, the lower the premium.

3. All urgent care provided at 0% co-pay.

4. Insurance companies will require patients to pay only a discounted portion of their selected co-pay, whatever that is, to hospitals or surgicenters for non-urgent care (to protect patients/consumers from huge bills).

5. Insurance companies will pay 100% of urgent care costs.

HOSPITALS & SURGICENTERS: New Rules

1. Triage and redirect E.R. patients for treatment or admission (only those that match the definition of Urgent/Catastrophic care). Direct all other patients to outreach clinics (not necessarily their own) or private care.

2. Post all fees (simplified and unbundled).

3. Bill appropriate fund for care that fits the appropriate definition and appropriately collect the adjusted co-pay or means-tested fee.

4. Leave Medicare alone for now.

5. Hospitals are required to set up and run outreach clinics for non-urgent care. All clinic fees are to be posted. Clinics will compete with other local hospital outreach clinics.

6. Pay all providers that work in their clinics their posted fees in full.

Item 6 above represents a benefit to providers. The provider (physician) who can charge only one fee (the fee posted) whenever he performs a specific service will earn more when he performs that same service in the hospital clinic setting. The provider will be paid that same fee by the hospital and will earn more by working in the hospital clinic than they would if they performed that service in their own office. (The provider incurs no overhead while working in the clinic.)

As a result, the hospital will have no problem recruiting medical talent to work in the clinic. Doctors will compete for these positions.

Details: Hospitals

A.   All hospitals will establish and run outreach clinics funded by the government via a specific formula. (Many already have.) This will provide for incredible savings by reducing the overloads in emergency rooms while at the same time providing appropriate and timely care to all people; not much different from what occurs now, but with much less waste of resources.

B.   These clinics will:

1.   Cover all specialties provided in the hospitals.

2.   Provide only non-urgent care.

3.   Care for all people with and without insurance. Co-pays apply if the patient has insurance. A means test will apply in place of a co-pay if the patient has no insurance.

4.   Provide a uniform **means test** to all patients so they pay according to what they can afford.

5.   Post their clinic fees for care like all other providers.

6. Charge the same fees as they posted and pay their doctors the fees that the doctors have posted.

7. Obligate providers and their staff to man these clinics. Since providers will be paid the same fees that they receive in their private practice (the fees that they posted), serving in these clinics will actually be desirable since the doctors will have less overhead.

C. The funding formula for these clinics can be a combination of:

1. Federal government funding, perhaps 50%.

2. Private insurance funding from a pool (like uninsured motorists) listed separately as an identified portion of everyone's premium, perhaps 10% labeled "uninsured care."

3. Charitable contributions from individuals and charitable organizations (fully tax deductible to donor).

4. State government. (All revenue sources designated by federal and state governments clearly identified and transparent)

D. Hospitals will now be able to redirect non-urgent care to their outreach clinics and unload their Emergency Rooms, and still make some profit from their outreach clinics. The outreach clinics will compete with each other.

E. Hospitals will collect only a predetermined discounted % of the patient-selected co-pay for all elective **inpatient** care.

F.   Hospital will bill all **uninsured patients** for in-house elective care based on a means test. (The same means test used in the outreach clinics.)

G.   Hospitals will bill all catastrophic care to the Catastrophic/Urgent Care Fund.

ATTORNEYS: New Rules

1. New national caps on pain and suffering.

2. Submit apparent frivolous LOST malpractice cases to the scrutiny of:

   a. Medical Peer Review Process

   b. Legal Peer Review Process

3. Be subjected to nominal penalties if all three processes (litigation and Peer Reviews) result in detrimental findings.

Details: Attorneys

Two pathways to real tort reform.

Fact 1: 30% of tests and care are originated by doctors who feel that they have to protect themselves from malpractice litigation.

Fact 11: 15% of providers as well as hospital fees are devoted to cover malpractice premiums.

Legislation 1: Caps on pain and suffering

Suggested awards from $250,000 to $450,000, with full reimbursement for true losses (wages, future care, etc.). This has been tried and has worked in every state where it has been tried.

Legislation 2: Penalties for filing frivolous malpractice lawsuits

1. Penalties not to exceed the true court costs (the waste of judicial time). Penalties are necessary; however, they must be fair.

2. Penalties to be split in reverse of contingency fee. (If the lawyer agrees upon a win, take 30% of the proceeds from the case. Then the lawyer is to pay 70% of the penalty and the patient pays 30% if the case is determined to be frivolous.)

3. The government is to create a new practical definition of frivolous which is different from the legal definition. Call it "Practical Frivolous" and let it be covered by the attorney's malpractice insurance:

   a. This new definition of frivolous is made up of three criteria. All three must be confirmed frivolous and all three must be in agreement with each other.

   Criteria #1: Lose the litigation. Had to be lost before a jury (no cause verdict).

   Criteria #2: Medical Peer Review Panel must find that the **provider was not at faul**t. Panel to be selected randomly from a pool, outside of the jurisdiction of the medical provider that was sued, and made up of three defense medical experts and three plaintiff medical experts and one randomly selected blindly from the same pool of an equal number of defense and plaintiff experts.

<u>Criteria #3</u>: Legal Peer Review made up of a panel of three randomly selected defense attorneys and three plaintiff attorneys and one selected blindly from the same pool of an equal number of defense and plaintiff attorneys. Each panel of attorneys to be selected from different jurisdictions and freshly appointed for each case. (Very similar to Medical Peer Review)

4. All expert witness testimony in all malpractice cases is to be published on the Internet and reviewed for scientific validity; review comments permitted on website.

   Periodic review of the comments to be undertaken by each state medical licensing board who will consider disciplinary action against expert witnesses if certain high threshold criteria are met and where truthful evidence-based and scientifically supported testimony is brought into question.

5. Lift prohibition against suing HMO's.

6. Substantial penalties should be imposed **for encouraging clients** to seek unnecessary medical treatment to enhance their probability of winning their litigation. Prosecution should be against the attorney as would any criminal case for conspiracy to commit insurance fraud.

PROVIDERS: New Rules

1. Post and annually update fees and qualifications on government website.

2. Agree to have one and only one fee for each service.

3. Disseminate fees upon request and post fees in the office.

4. Collect co-pays or means-tested fees from all patients.

5. Bill all urgent/catastrophic care to the appropriate pool (no co-pay). You will be paid 100% of your fee every time.

6. Be available and affirm the second opinion requirement when indicated.

Details: Providers—doctors, hospitals, physical therapists, chiropractors, etc. (all providers)

A. Require **all providers** of medical services to:

1. Post all of their fees and charge only those fees to all patients and all payers (using descriptions and current codes).

Robert Dennis, MD

a. Make all fees easy to understand. (Like all other commodities)

b. Agree to have one and only one fee for each service.

c. Describe all fees in pamphlets, faxes, waiting room, posters, websites, etc. (all fees must be in a meaningful order of frequency).

d. Describe all fees in the order of their most common services to their least common services.

e. Post the single most appropriate, fair, reasonable, and realistic fee that they must accept for that given service and that they expect to be paid each time they perform that service regardless of who they bill or who ends up paying. (No one will set these fees but them.) Each provider will then quickly adjust to the true market forces of supply and demand.

The law of supply and demand will quickly take over.

f. Agree to provide their fees to all patients at all times and most importantly before their appointment and require signature of the patient (like HIPPA).

g. Utilize already established CPT codes with the same unbundling rules that currently apply.

h. Re-affirm or change their fees on an annual basis.

i. Understand all laws to end price fixings as it affects them and expect to be prosecuted if found guilty.

2. Post their qualifications: credentials, malpractice history, practice history, most frequently performed procedures, complication rate, etc.

3. Post fees and qualifications on uniform, sortable websites to be maintained by the government.

4. Be responsible to verify and update their information annually.

5. Expect to be prosecuted for conspiracy to commit insurance fraud in cases where practice patterns reflect abuse or excessive treatment, particularly when litigation or entitlement programs are liable for medical bills. (Enhanced prosecution of medical, legal mills.)

6. Bill all care defined to be catastrophic care to catastrophic pool.

This plan will eliminate pre-authorization/precertification and referrals, along with all the bureaucracy and costs associated.

Robert Dennis, MD

PATIENTS: New Rules

Patients will be expected to:

1. Shop insurance policies based on only two variable parameters:

   a. Amount of co-pay (% of fees)

   b. Dollar amount of threshold for second opinion (the lower the threshold, the lower the premium)

2. Pay their share of the co-pay or means test for every piece of elective care (skin in the game).

3. Shop and purchase all elective medical care based on transparent and easily available cost and quality parameters.

4. If they have no insurance, select a hospital-run outreach clinic and be means tested for all elective care (the means test could require the patient to pay as little as 0.5% or 0% of all care).

5. Obtain and abide by the required second opinions.

Details: Patients (Below age 65)

A. Will be **required** to obtain second opinions for all non-urgent procedures over a certain amount; with no restrictions on a patient switching doctors. (Good for patients, good for doctors and good for the system.)

   1. Patients to select the second opinion doctor for consultation in the same way and for the same posted fee as the patient selected the first doctor.

   2. Patients select their second opinion threshold amount when they purchase their insurance. This will vary according to their choice. (The higher the threshold, the higher the premium; the lower the threshold amount they choose, the lower their insurance premium.) Insurance companies will want to encourage second opinions as a means of lowering their costs.

B. Shop for cost and quality to save their own money (via co-pay) in the same way as they would shop for any other item; by becoming knowledgeable and shopping price vs. quality (all of which is now readily available to them and will lower costs enormously).

C. Complete and sign a living will to address how they wish to be treated.

   1. A living will is a requirement. Generic wills are to be offered at a fixed minimal cost or free.

   2. The will describes a variety of circumstances and options regarding heroic methods of extending life under a number of circumstances (much as they do now).

Robert Dennis, MD

3. They will include options for organ donation if they so desire. Their personal living will can be changed and re-signed in the same way they are now.

4. Family and estates will be responsible for outstanding bills, no differently than they are today.

5. A generic will, generally agreed upon and well written, will apply as a default "living will" for all those who have not signed their own personal will.

6. Living wills will be readily available to health care providers via the Internet and other forms of communication, much as they are today utilizing POLST (Practitioner Orders for Life-Sustaining Treatment).

Summary: The need for pre-authorizations/precertifications, primary care referrals, as well as all other paperwork and delays will be eliminated. This will in turn eliminate the bureaucracy and associated costs. All catastrophic care will be billed to the catastrophic fund with 0% co-pay to the patient. All urgent care will be paid for by their insurance company via their contribution to the Urgent Care Fund with 0% co-pay to the patient.

This chapter has summarized the new obligations and responsibilities of each of the six participants. Each were previously considered to be separate cost centers or generators of layered fees. By redefining the roles of all six, the cost of the entire conglomerate of healthcare goods and services will be dramatically reduced.

We can anticipate enormous resistance to change. Each stakeholder is expected to vigorously object and find endless reasons why this dramatic new concept can't work. However, when one looks at it from an overview it is most simple and nothing more than the way it would have evolved had it not been for the political interference of each of the six participants. The current crisis is the result of the layered bureaucracy created over time. We believe it is time to correct these distortions.

Chapter 11: Funding: Tax Reductions, Not Increases

This may be hard for industry experts to fathom. One can understand the effect that 40 years of piled on paperwork and bureaucratic administration has had on all of us.

However, all a person needs do is add up the current **total** healthcare expenditure which will now include **an additional $70 billion** of more government administrative workers in the IRS and other agencies to just administer the Affordable Care Act. Add to that the billions of dollars spent by insurance carriers and providers just to deal with bureaucratic paperwork issues. Then, add to that the billions of dollars asked to support medical care which includes all the Medicaid programs as well as all the annual insurance premiums paid into the insurance companies.

Excluding Medicare and removing the recently added new taxes from Obamacare, the medical budget remaining to fund the Informed Health Plan Act (IHPA) is still in the trillions. This will be more than enough resources to totally fund all aspects of urgent and uninsured care described in this program, and taxes will be able to be substantially reduced. Although this may sound unrealistic, please appreciate the impact that this concept will have on the delivery of healthcare across this country.

Nothing described thus far should initially apply to Medicare which remains outside of the system at least until the system is proven successful and all the bugs worked out. Medicare and all Medicare recipients are therefore excluded.

Also, the redundant and overly expensive state programs that provide a completely separate health care system under the Worker's Compensation and No-Fault Laws in each state should be temporarily excluded. However in the future, as the system proves itself, these two additional redundant and excessive programs can later ultimately be folded into and be included in the Informed Health Plan Act (IHPA).

With that as the backdrop, we can go forward to understand exactly how easy it will be to redirect those funds into a single, simple plan that will provide medical care for everyone by using the market system within the elective portion, thereby reducing the cost over the entire system. By that we mean the current system's redundant, wasteful and layered bureaucracy that currently manages to fund all the acute and catastrophic care that is being provided at this very moment. Therefore, no additional funding sources will actually be necessary to pay for the acute care portion of this program. We are reasonably sure that actuaries will substantiate this statement. Let's look at how this plan can be funded in a very transparent and simple fashion.

Robert Dennis, MD

Chapter 12: Funding Urgent Care/ Catastrophic Care

INFORMED Health Plan Provides For All Health Needs

Two Pools of Funds

**All Health Care is Paid for
From One of These Two Pools**

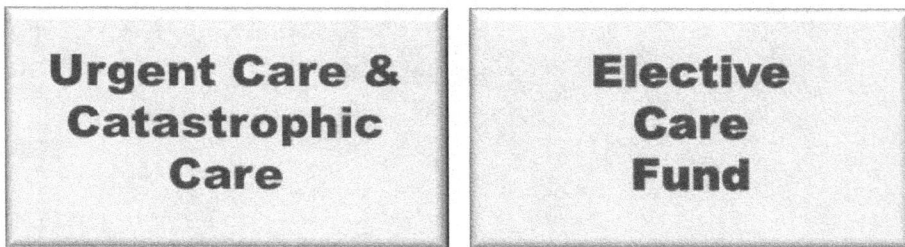

Urgent Care & Catastrophic Care	**Elective Care Fund**

Essentially there are two pools of funds. They are divided along the lines of the definitions previously discussed. Each pool is funded slightly differently. If the provider is providing urgent care, he bills one central fund which represents the pool of monies from several sources. He bills the fees that he has posted for the procedures that he has described. He can bill no more or no less. When he performs a service defined within the catastrophic definition, he bills the same posted fee to the catastrophic fund and does not collect the co-pay from the patient.

When the patient receives care defined as catastrophic or urgent care, no second opinion threshold applies and they are certainly not going to be asked to pay any co-pay. The funding derives as follows:

How is the Urgent/Catastrophic Pool Funded?

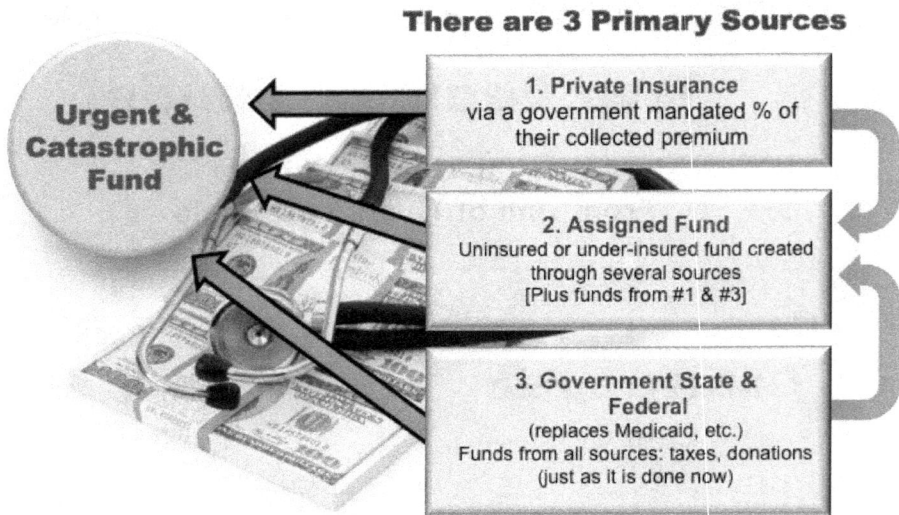

There are 3 Primary Sources

Urgent & Catastrophic Fund

1. Private Insurance via a government mandated % of their collected premium

2. Assigned Fund
Uninsured or under-insured fund created through several sources
[Plus funds from #1 & #3]

3. Government State & Federal
(replaces Medicaid, etc.)
Funds from all sources: taxes, donations
(just as it is done now)

The funding sources for urgent care are actually very similar to the way that urgent care is funded today. These funds are currently more than adequate.

Today, if an uninsured person or even a foreign guest gets hit by a truck the sources of funding include the same Medicaid government funding that currently provides care to that patient. Certainly, a portion of that patient's care is covered by the hospital's over-billing of many private patients which unfortunately creates even more distortion of who's paying for what. Private premiums presently pay part of the care for the uninsured even now.

The previous diagram simply spells this out very clearly. The annual invoices for private insurance premiums will, quite transparently, spell it out even better as illustrated below:

How are Private Insurance Premiums Calculated by Companies?

Each company is notified annually by the government as to how much is required of their premium dollar to help fund the:

1. Uninsured or underinsured fund (x% of premium)
2. UC Fund (x% of premium)
   These %'s will vary annually but will be the same for all insurance companies

Insurance bill to each insured looks like this

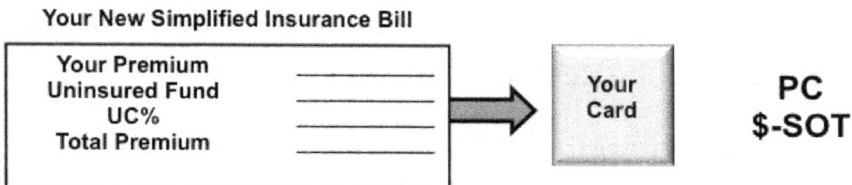

Your New Simplified Insurance Bill

Your Premium	_____
Uninsured Fund	_____
UC%	_____
Total Premium	_____

→ Your Card   PC $-SOT

If you look at this insurance premium invoice statement you will see only three line items. This is the ultimate in transparency.

Each insurance company will be advised at the beginning of each year by the government actuaries, how much of the **uninsured burden** the private sector will be asked to cover. Their company will have to bear a proportional amount of the total. In a similar fashion, the government actuaries will inform the private sector as to how much they will have to bear to cover the **urgent care/catastrophic fund**. Each private company will be assessed proportionally.

Each insurance company will then divide that amount up over the number of their insureds and that figure will be printed on your monthly invoice. Funding does not get more transparent than that!

These government assessments will be distributed evenly across all the private insurance companies and will be the total contribution needed to fund those specific pools after all government funds have already been absorbed within those categories.

Needless to say, the individual's insurance premium statement will clearly itemize that portion of the total premium that has been assigned to them via the two government pools, as well the amount that they are actually paying for the type of insurance that they had selected. That portion will depend on the specific percent co-pay "PC" and "SOT" that the individual selected. This will be described in later chapters.

It is important to appreciate that the Urgent Care Fund will completely and fully cover the privately insured consumers in the exact same way that it covers the urgent care of the poor, underinsured and uninsured. Not by what or who paid the premiums, but by the **definition**. The private insurance companies are completely free of those costs for their insured.

Chapter 13: Elective Care Funding

There are only two variables to keep in mind when a person obtains insurance coverage for elective care: the percent co-pay and the second opinion threshold (SOT). Private insurance can be purchased on the Internet. The insurance companies will compete but each is free to charge whatever premium they wish based on just these two variables. The consumer will make the final decision as to what he or she wishes to purchase and how much they wish to pay.

In a similar way, depending on income, anyone can purchase or be assigned government-sponsored coverage based on the same two variables. The person's accompanying card simply provides the basic information to the provider and represents the criteria of the two variables that apply to any given patient.

It is just that simple.

How is the Elective Pool Funded?

There are 3 Primary Sources

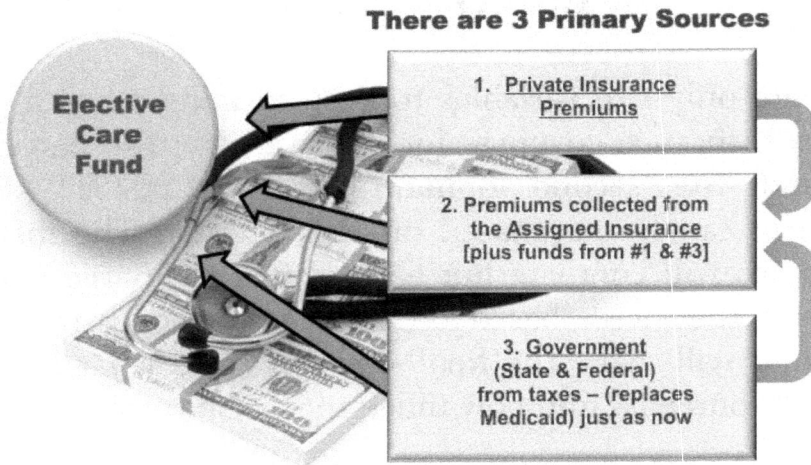

Elective Care Fund

1. <u>Private Insurance Premiums</u>

2. Premiums collected from the <u>Assigned Insurance</u> [plus funds from #1 & #3]

3. <u>Government</u> (State & Federal) from taxes – (replaces Medicaid) just as now

When providers offer treatment that is defined as elective care they bill their posted fee to either the insurance company or to the elective care fund. They must bill the patient the percent co-pay described on the patient's insurance card. The amount that the provider bills the fund or the insurance carrier is of course minus whatever he or she collected from the patient. The physician is obligated to collect the percent co-pay from the patient. The patient's insurance card (which is to be used only for elective care) will simply describe the three key pieces of information required by the provider:

1. The name and address of the payor (insurance company or elective care fund)

2. The percent co-pay

3. The second opinion threshold (SOT)

Every person can obtain an insurance card which will provide him with access to elective care! The next question that needs to be answered is: how does a person obtain an insurance card? There are three options:

Option #1:

Purchase insurance from the government-managed insurance website.

Can Everyone Obtain a Healthcare Card?
There are Three Options!
Option #1
Private Insurance Card

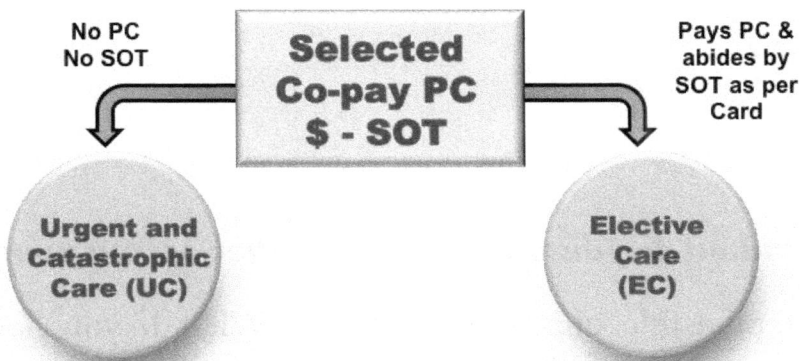

No PC
No SOT

Selected
Co-pay PC
$ - SOT

Pays PC &
abides by
SOT as per
Card

Urgent and
Catastrophic
Care (UC)

Elective
Care
(EC)

23

Option #2:

For low-income individuals—a means-tested card from their hospital outreach clinic.

Can Everyone Obtain a Healthcare Card?
There are Three Options!

Option #2
Means Tested Card

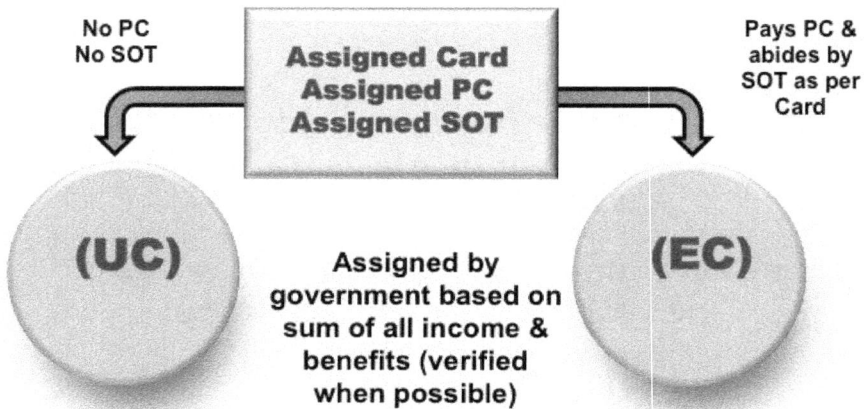

No PC
No SOT

Assigned Card
Assigned PC
Assigned SOT

Pays PC &
abides by
SOT as per
Card

(UC)

Assigned by
government based on
sum of all income &
benefits (verified
when possible)

(EC)

25

Option #3:

An individual decides not to select either option #1 or #2.

The next plausible question would be: What if you had no
insurance card? To fully understand the implications of that
question please keep in mind that the free market competition
will have lowered the providers' fees to real or actual market
value. This means that the posted fees will no longer be
astronomical but rather realistic and balanced by the
competition and the real costs, giving providers fair profit with
minimal overhead.

Can Everyone Obtain a Healthcare Card?
There are Three Options!
Option #3

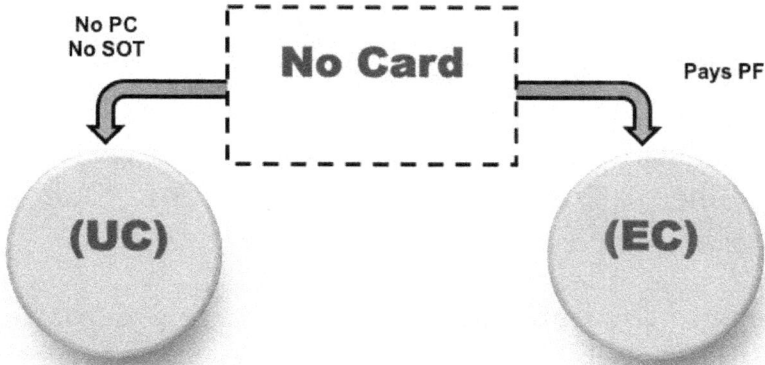

However, even if an individual chooses not to select any of the options, they will still be able to fully access both urgent and elective care at low and realistic fees brought down to actual market value because of the Informed Health Plan Act.

And What if You Have No Card?
How Would You Access Elective Care?

Option #3

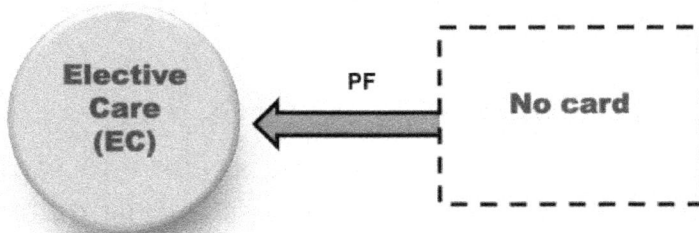

Rich or Poor, You Can Choose Not to Purchase Insurance
OR
Not to Even Apply for an Assigned Card

Irrespective of how the consumer does or doesn't obtain coverage, the providers' fees would be transparent and available for all to see and providers would not be permitted to charge more than that fee.

> **Summary:** Elective care is billed to the insurer minus the percent co-pay in Option #1, and in Option #2, from the uninsured fund, according to the rules. In Option #3, the full provider fee would be billed to the patient who chose not to obtain any insurance.
>
> Despite the pathway, IHPA lowers fees across all options and permits full access for everyone. Urgent care is available for all members of society, and even those with no insurance card are fully served because all such bills for urgent care are billed directly to the urgent care fund.

Regardless of which of the three options are used to obtain an insurance card for elective care, there are no restrictions on what care you can seek. In addition, since there are no provider networks, there are no restrictions on the providers that you can seek. Finally, there are no denials, penalties, necessary referrals or bureaucratic algorithms that will affect your access to elective medical care.

It was previously stated that one of the key government responsibilities was to create an actuarial curve to provide for a means-tested insurance card and access to hospital outreach clinics to guarantee that care will be provided to all members of society.

Does everyone have to buy insurance?

Are there penalties to the individual or employer if you choose not to buy insurance?

The answer to these two questions is an absolute. unequivocal "No!!"

WITH INSURANCE

Who Does The Provider Bill?
What Does the Provider Charge?

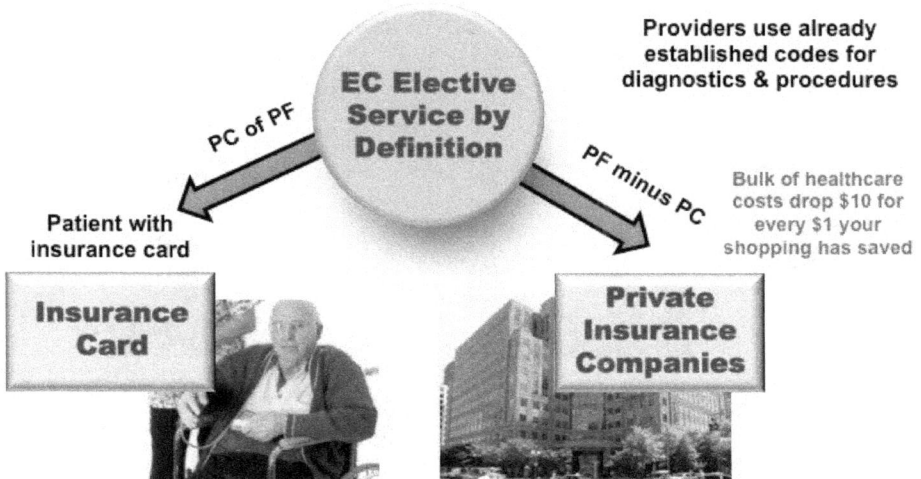

PC of PF

PF minus PC

EC Elective Service by Definition

Providers use already established codes for diagnostics & procedures

Patient with insurance card

Bulk of healthcare costs drop $10 for every $1 your shopping has saved

Insurance Card

Private Insurance Companies

WITHOUT INSURANCE

Low income or no income patients are provided with a means-tested insurance card provided by the Government at a hospital intake desk.

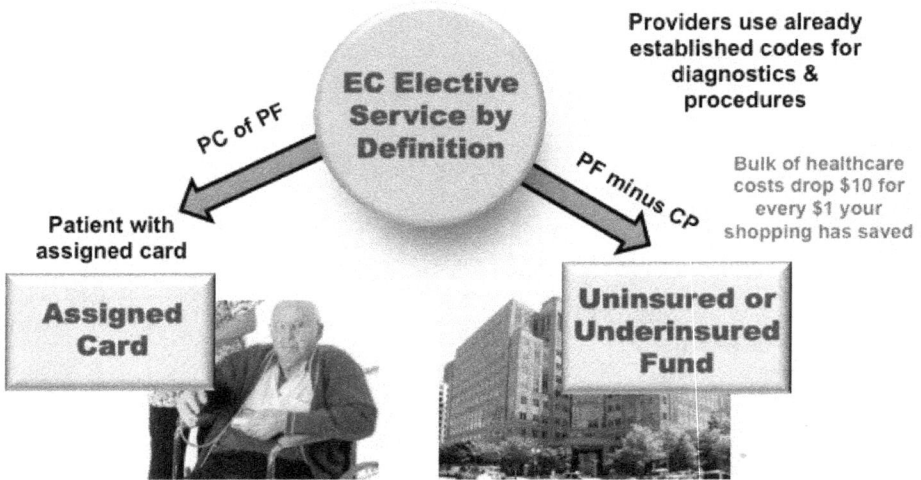

Who Does The Provider Bill?
& What Does the Provider Charge?

EC Elective Service by Definition

PC of PF

PF minus CP

Providers use already established codes for diagnostics & procedures

Bulk of healthcare costs drop $10 for every $1 your shopping has saved

Patient with assigned card

Assigned Card

Uninsured or Underinsured Fund

With No Card

(Patient has no insurance and no insurance card but wishes ELECTIVE CARE.)

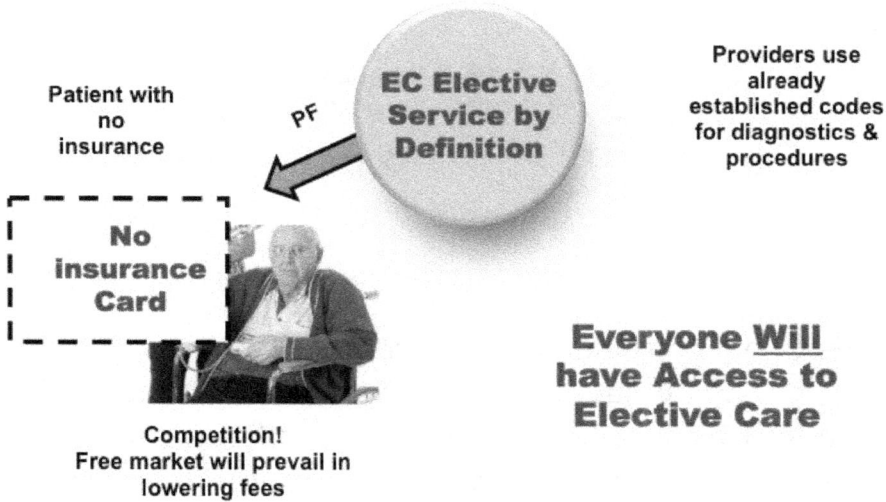

Who Does The Provider Bill?
& What Does the Provider Charge?

Patient with no insurance

PF

EC Elective Service by Definition

Providers use already established codes for diagnostics & procedures

No insurance Card

Everyone **Will** have Access to Elective Care

Competition!
Free market will prevail in lowering fees

Where Do Patients Access Elective Care?

Elective Care
Doctors' Offices
Hospital Outreach Clinics
Drug Stores
Hospitals
Surgicenters
Etc.

ER Triage nurse applies definitions for treatment for admission or treatment.

(Only UC is to be treated in ERs.)

ER providers must send patients who require only EC to Hospital Outreach Clinics or Private Doctors

**What can these providers charge?
ONLY THEIR POSTED FEES
Free Market Will Work Over Short Time**

If a patient goes to the emergency room for the first time with a non-urgent issue such as a cold, once the triage nurse or physician affirms that the patient is not suffering from a life-threatening condition, they are required to then refer the patient to the hospital outreach clinic the following day, in the exact same manner that they would refer a patient to a private physician. This is not different than before except that the new definitions prohibit the ER physician from beginning to treat any patient suffering from a non-urgent condition.

By the time the patient appears in the emergency room for a second time with the same non-urgent condition they would have or should have already been provided with a means-tested insurance card at the same ER intake desk and this time referred directly to the hospital outreach clinic. These new definitions will therefore ultimately, reduce the inappropriate

Robert Dennis, MD

use of the emergency room by the uninsured or for that matter even by the insured patient. Again, the system will experience a marked cost reduction.

Chapter 14: Accessing and Funding Urgent Care

Finally, free health care for all and the funding mechanism to support it!

This plan establishes a transparent funding structure that provides for free care for the entire population for any and all treatments related to any and all life- or limb-threatening care, i.e. URGENT CARE (non-elective by definition). No longer will there be cases of an impoverished mother unable to purchase insulin for her diabetic daughter. No longer will we question how the medical care is provided for an impoverished soul who gets hit by a truck.

Please recall, we previously discussed that when care is provided for life-threatening or limb-threatening defined conditions, the provider of that care still must bill only what he or she posted as the accepted fee and cannot bill the patient for any co-pay, nor is the patient bound to their insurance contract to obtain second opinions (which may be required for elective care).

The proper billing path is decided when the diagnosis is made. Currently no patient is treated without a diagnosis being attached to the billing invoice. No procedure is billed without a CPT code. This new concept does not change that requirement in any way.

Patients initially access emergency care in a hospital or urgent care setting. (No different than is done currently.) Sometimes patients are told that they might have a life-threatening condition in the doctor's office.

No matter where such a diagnosis is made, a life- or limb-threatening condition is paid for via the appropriate funded pool for as long as the patient is being treated for that particular condition. It is important to add that in the current system of medical coding the diagnosis is already tied to the various procedures appropriate for treatment of that specific diagnosis. This already functioning apparatus remains intact and will be fully utilized in this IHPA.

Can Everyone Access Urgent/ Catastrophic Care? Yes! Everyone Rich & Poor

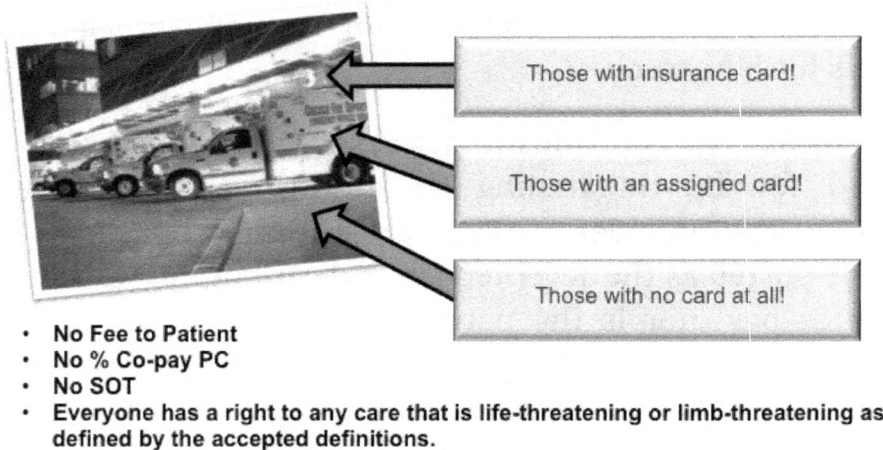

Those with insurance card!

Those with an assigned card!

Those with no card at all!

- • No Fee to Patient
- • No % Co-pay PC
- • No SOT
- • Everyone has a right to any care that is life-threatening or limb-threatening as defined by the accepted definitions.

31

There will be no change in the location or manner in which a patient receives urgent care.

Where Do Patients Access Elective Care?

Elective Care
Doctors' Offices
Hospital Outreach Clinics
Drug Stores
Hospitals
Surgicenters
Etc.

ER Triage nurse applies definitions for treatment for admission or treatment.

(Only UC is to be treated in ERs.)

ER providers must send patients who require only EC to Hospital Outreach Clinics or Private Doctors

What can these providers charge?
ONLY THEIR POSTED FEES
Free Market Will Work Over Short Time

All urgent care is billed directly to the urgent care fund. It is important to note that any attempts to misleadingly categorize certain treatments as urgent (which could be a source of fraud and abuse) would be quickly and easily nipped in the bud because all the bills are sent to a single central office and can easily be monitored and addressed at that point.

Who Does the Provider Bill?
What Does the Provider Charge?

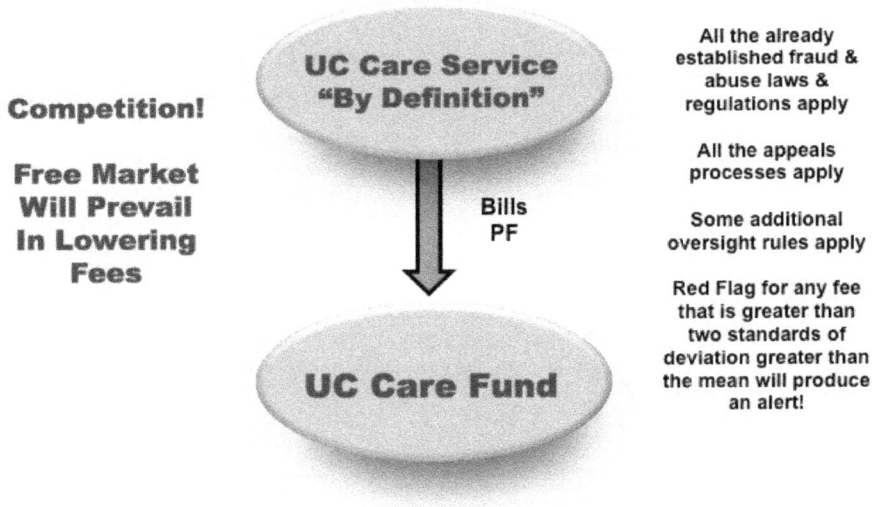

UC Care Service "By Definition"

All the already established fraud & abuse laws & regulations apply

All the appeals processes apply

Competition!

Free Market Will Prevail In Lowering Fees

Bills
PF

Some additional oversight rules apply

Red Flag for any fee that is greater than two standards of deviation greater than the mean will produce an alert!

UC Care Fund

In this way the best possible treatment, equal for all, both the rich and the poor, is fully available to our entire society with or without insurance cards, with or without insurance, with or without even a means-tested card.

Recap from previous chapters:

Examples of life-threatening and limb-threatening care:

- Catastrophic care
- Cancer care
- Acute cardiac care, including cardiac catheterization, stents, angioplasties, acute pulmonary care
- Fracture care
- Anything that threatens life or limb either in the short-term or long-term or anything, the treatment of which if delayed, might jeopardize life or limb.

How is the Urgent/Catastrophic Pool Funded?

There are 3 Primary Sources

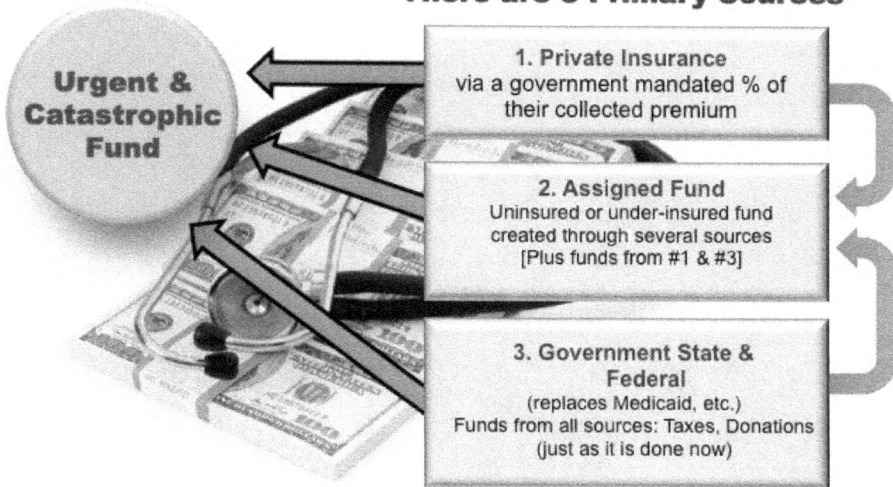

Urgent & Catastrophic Fund

1. Private Insurance
via a government mandated % of their collected premium

2. Assigned Fund
Uninsured or under-insured fund created through several sources
[Plus funds from #1 & #3]

3. Government State & Federal
(replaces Medicaid, etc.)
Funds from all sources: Taxes, Donations
(just as it is done now)

Robert Dennis, MD

Chapter 15: Review and Further Details

1. All patients have skin in the game for all elective care.

2. All urgent care is free to the rich and poor.

3. Anyone can go to any willing licensed provider in any state (no networks).

4. Providers get their full fee and competition will control prices.

5. Paperwork, bureaucracy, and administrative costs will be minimized.

6. Government has an appropriate role (not too big or too small).

7. Fraud and abuse will be punished severely (central locations receive all bills).

8. The SOT replaces billions of dollars of bureaucracy. (Second opinions for EC is beneficial and doesn't hurt anyone. It better informs us all).

9. Patients can shop quality and cost as easily as they can shop for a TV. The mystery veil is removed. The separation of cost from care is removed as it applies to elective care.

10. Patients shop for providers and insurance the same way.

Everything that has been discussed to this point was specifically and exclusively silent on some key issues:

1. All insurances can be sold across state lines. There are no networks. Any patient/consumer can go to

any "willing provider" in any state.

2. There are no pre-existing conditions mentioned because in this plan there are no pre-existing conditions that would affect a patient's/consumer's ability to purchase insurance. This is purposely not mentioned because, as you will see, pre-existing conditions have no place in, nor are even considered in the pricing of insurance premiums.

3. Children (of the age of 26 and even beyond) remaining at home with their parents can be added to their parents' insurance contract.

4. There are no employer mandates or penalties imposed upon the individual or the employer (there doesn't need to be in a free market system).

5. There are no individual subsidies needed, or extra and hidden taxes in this system (there doesn't need to be any in a competitive market system).

6. No need to hire thousands of additional administrators or create new government departments. Forget the $70 billion estimated and new bureaucratic costs that provide no medical benefit to any person recently announced to implement Obamacare.

7. No need to expand the IRS to collect any new taxes.

8. Medical savings plans will be expanded and are part of the IHPA.

9. There are no rationing committees.

10. There is no need to grant waivers to special groups.

Chapter 16: Behind the Scenes Actuaries Are Hard at Work

Informed Health Plan Behind The Scenes

How Does It Really Work?

Here is how it really works. This complex chapter will be presented in the order that best addresses the questions that have arisen by now. The reader is asked to suspend the requirement for full comprehension until after all the unique aspects of the program have been reviewed and all the pieces of the puzzle are re-assembled.

Both at the insurance companies and in Washington, actuarial expertise is required to make sure appropriate funding is provided and directed in the correct manner.

The calculations under IHPA will be much simpler than they are today and based on dramatically different parameters. There are only two parameters to be measured. These come down to a simple curve on a graph based on actuarial fundamentals. Your full attention will be needed here to understand the simplicity of this new concept.

The only two variables that have to be calculated and that go on to an insurance card are the:

PC and SOT

How Do Insurance Companies and Government Means Tested Formulas Set the Only Two Variables in the System?

PC & SOT

The same way they do now, by targeting their markets and using actual calculations.

How do insurance companies figure out their premiums?

Behind The Scenes
Actuaries are hard at work!

Just as they are now!

First they determine the premium that would be related to the percent co-pay (PC) they wish to offer their customers. As below:

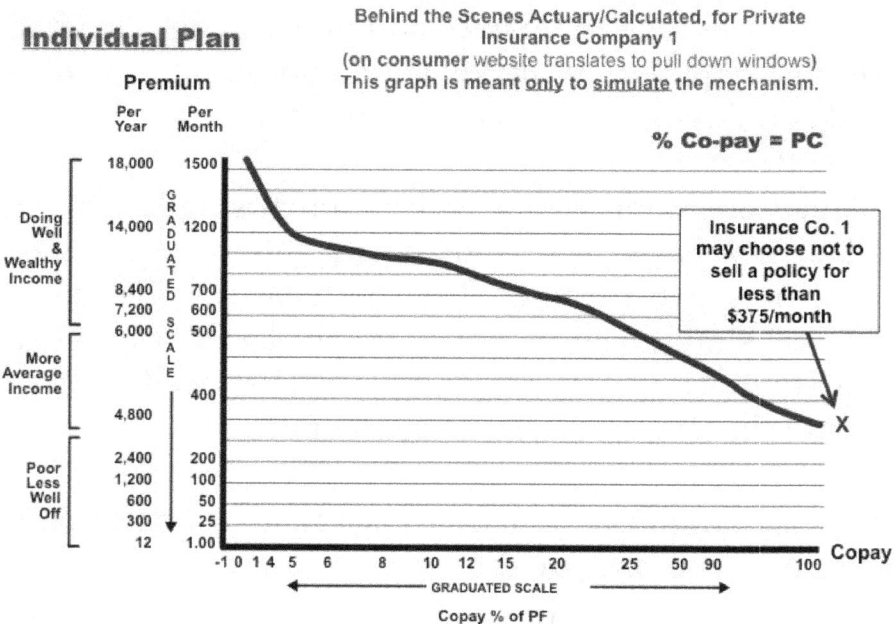

Behind the Scenes Actuary/Calculated, for Private Insurance Company 1
(on consumer website translates to pull down windows)
This graph is meant only to simulate the mechanism.

Individual Plan

% Co-pay = PC

Insurance Co. 1 may choose not to sell a policy for less than $375/month

The higher the premium that the consumer chooses, the lower the percent co-pay and vice versa; the lower the percent co-pay is chosen by the consumer, the higher will be the premium.

Then they would figure out the second opinion threshold (SOT) that they wish to offer their customers for a given premium. As below:

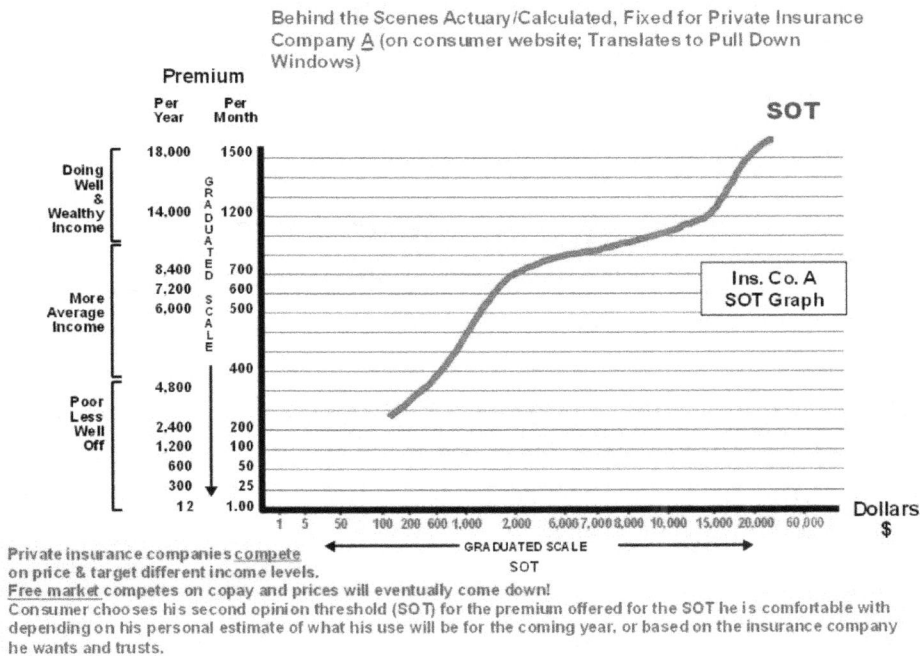

Behind the Scenes Actuary/Calculated, Fixed for Private Insurance Company A (on consumer website; Translates to Pull Down Windows)

Private insurance companies compete on price & target different income levels.
Free market competes on copay and prices will eventually come down!
Consumer chooses his second opinion threshold (SOT) for the premium offered for the SOT he is comfortable with depending on his personal estimate of what his use will be for the coming year, or based on the insurance company he wants and trusts.

The higher the premium that the consumer chooses, the higher will be the threshold (high SOT) that requires a second opinion and vice versa; the lower the threshold is that triggers the need for a second opinion (low SOT) the lower the premium.

The process requires that each insurance company targets their potential customers by income level and where they wish to be in the marketplace. Insurance Company A's graph might look like this:

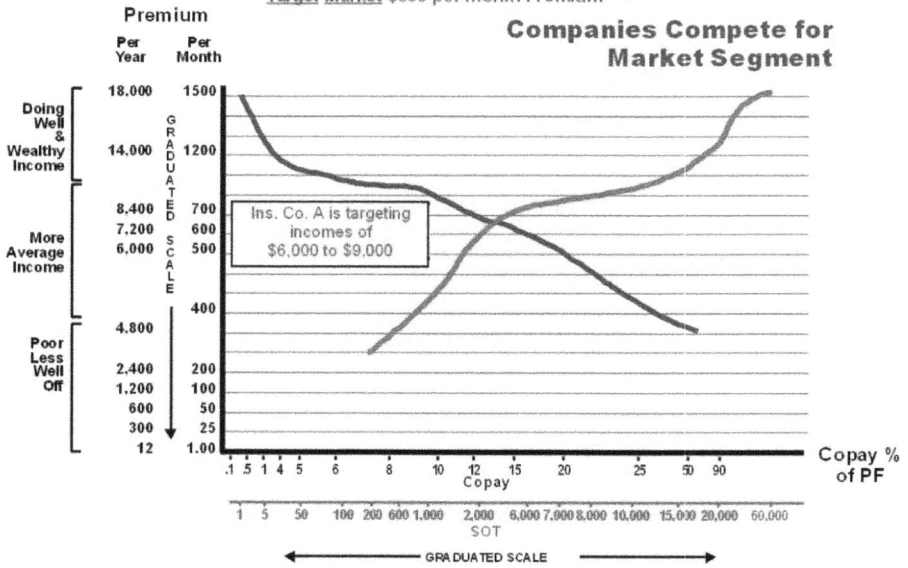

This simply means that Insurance Company A considers their ideal market, households that earn slightly more than the average income and can afford a premium of $6,000 to $8,000 per year, and would consider a policy that had between a 10% to 20% co-pay.

They also calculated that their target market would be interested in a SOT range between $1,800 and $6,000. The premium that they would charge for those two variables that a customer may select would come right off of this simple two-parameter, actuarially generated chart, specifically designed for and by Insurance Company A to capture a specific portion of the private insurance market.

Insurance Company A would then convert this graph to drop-

Robert Dennis, MD

down windows on a simple website that would compete with other insurance carriers for the same or different segments of the market. The entire insurance industry would thereby become simplified, totally transparent, bureaucratically almost weightless, no longer in control of your healthcare, no longer between you and your physician, and fully competitive in the marketplace.

Meanwhile, Insurance Company B may target households with incomes that were willing to pay between $5,000 and $7,000 per year and accept % co-pay of 12-to-15% and an SOT of $2,000-to-$4,000.

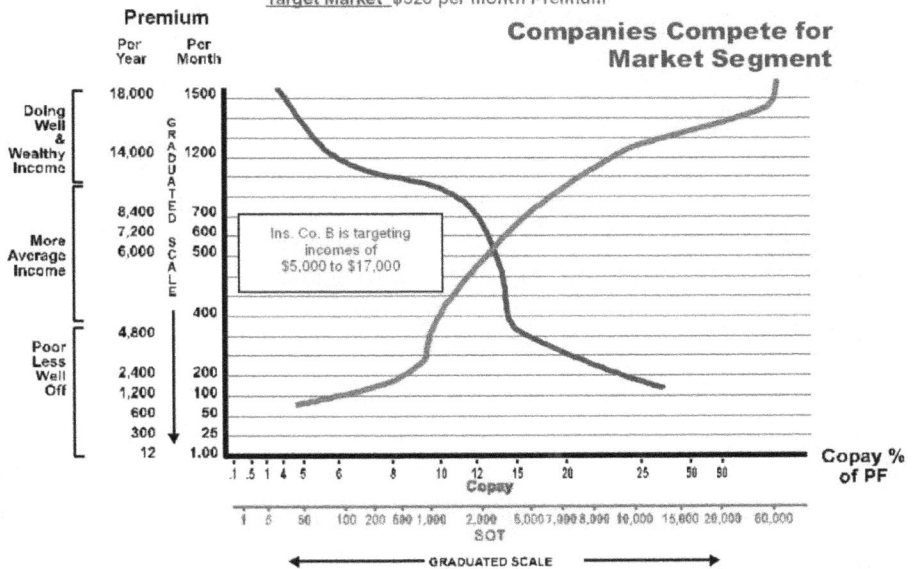

Individual Plan

Behind the Scenes Actuary/Calculated, Fixed for Private Insurance Combination of Each Company's CP and SOT (consumer website; will see this as pull down windows) Comparing Company B Target Market $520 per month Premium

Premium

Per Year / Per Month

Companies Compete for Market Segment

GRADUATED SCALE

Doing Well & Wealthy Income

More Average Income

Poor Less Well Off

Ins. Co. B is targeting incomes of $5,000 to $17,000

18,000 / 1500
14,000 / 1200
8,400 / 700
7,200 / 600
6,000 / 500
400
4,800
2,400 / 200
1,200 / 100
600 / 50
300 / 25
12 / 1.00

.1 .5 1 4 5   6   8   10 12 15   20   25 50 90
Copay

Copay % of PF

1 5 50 100 200 500 1,000 2,000 5,000 7,000 8,000 10,000 15,000 20,000 60,000
SOT

GRADUATED SCALE

Other insurance companies would produce similar graphs that may appear like this behind the scenes:

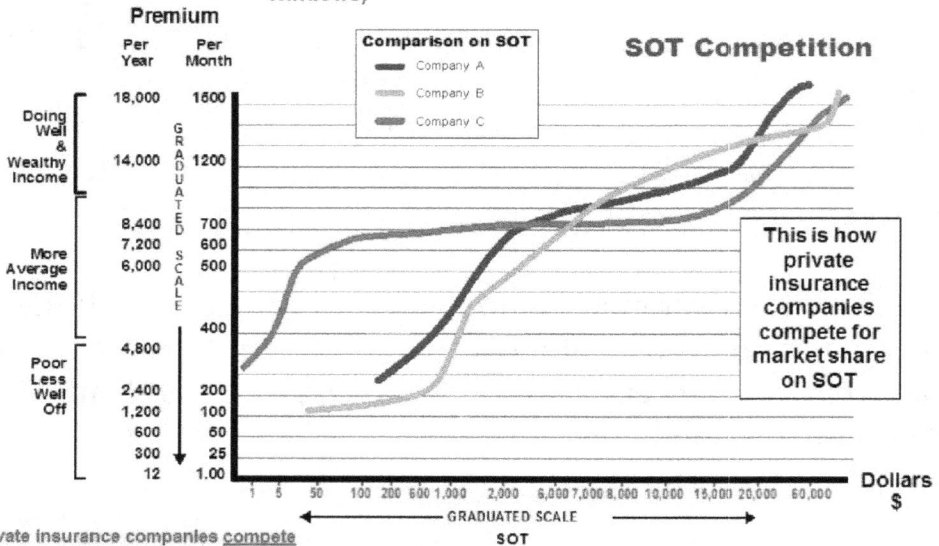

Individual Plan

Behind the Scenes Actuary/Calculated, Fixed for Private Insurance Companies (on consumer website; Translates to Pull Down Windows)

Premium

	Per Year	Per Month
Doing Well & Wealthy Income	18,000	1600
	14,000	1200
More Average Income	8,400	700
	7,200	600
	6,000	500
	4,800	400
Poor Less Well Off	2,400	200
	1,200	100
	600	50
	300	25
	12	1.00

GRADUATED SCALE

Comparison on SOT
- Company A
- Company B
- Company C

SOT Competition

This is how private insurance companies compete for market share on SOT

Dollars $

GRADUATED SCALE
SOT

Private insurance companies compete on price & target different income levels.
Free market competes on copay and prices will eventually come down!
Consumer chooses his second opinion threshold (SOT) for the premium offered for the SOT he is comfortable with depending on his personal estimate of what his use will be for the coming year, or based on the insurance company he wants and trusts.

The shape and slope of these curves presented by each of the insurance carriers competing for their market share represent the total picture of the premiums being offered to the consumer. It is not any more complicated than that! The carriers will compete in an open and transparent marketplace.

The webpage representation where the insurance companies actually compete in the marketplace would be presented to the public as no more than drop down box/user-friendly conversion of the underlying actuary curves produced and would look like this to the consumer purchasing insurance:

User Friendly Window for Consumer Insurance.
How Do Patients Select Insurance?

Percent Copay (PC)	Second Opinion Threshold (SOT)	Zip Code	Compare Price
Consumer Selects	Consumer Selects		
15% (PC)	$1,000 (SOT)	07757	$300/month Ins. Company A $200/month Ins. Company B $150/month Ins. Company C x x x x Ins. Co. D - Not Available in that price range

(Full Disclaimer: These graphs and estimates are just that—
rough estimates provided in order to give the reader an idea as
to how this plan actually operates behind the scenes. We do
not claim to be actuaries and these numbers and data are
fictitious and for illustrative purposes only.)

Robert Dennis, MD

Chapter 17: The Government's Role in This Free-Market System

Government actuaries provide insurance cards for elective care to patients who cannot afford private insurance, or can afford private insurance but choose the government plan instead for whatever reason.

The government plan is specifically designed to be very unattractive for wealthy households. Actuarial yet simple management of the slope of the curve is all that is required. The same graph, by its very design, provides a very fair and appropriate insurance plan for the uninsured or underinsured for elective care. It's no more complicated than that!

From this single simple curve (ZIP Code adjusted) and available at every hospital intake desk, low income households can be easily provided with insurance coverage for all elective care.

Assigned Care:

Behind the scenes actuaries are hard at work identifying income levels that qualify for specific assigned parameters of PC & SOT.

The Means Test sets up a simple and uniform mechanism to provide an assigned card to rich & poor alike.

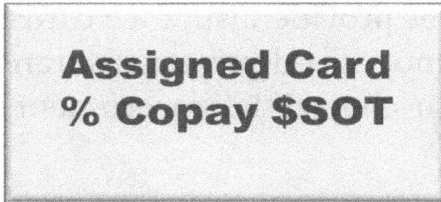

```
Assigned Card
% Copay $SOT
```

Anyone and everyone is eligible for an assigned card if they so choose. The rich, the poor, and the newly welcomed visitors to our country can obtain a card. It is a pure function of their income. Income verification is required. Even if they make $2000 a year from picking fruit or mowing lawns and do not file taxes or if they make a poverty level income or millions of dollars, it doesn't matter. If they can show some proof of what their income is, either a high or low or zero, any and all of us will be able to obtain a government-issued assigned card.

Most of us who could afford insurance will find that the private market will charge us less and give us more than the assigned government card. But that is totally up to the individual. Yes, the government will compete with the private market but the private market will not want to target the low income brackets that the government program will be happy to cover.

Please remember that this plan replaces Medicaid and all the funding that would normally be directed through the Medicaid program. All of that funding would now be redirected to this new plan—the assigned card program. The actuarial-designed government plan may look like this:

How Does The Government Go About Assigning A Card Based On Income?

By utilizing a simple, actuary-generated graph. This graph is uniform across the country and varies only by zip code.
This means test favors lower incomes but also permits anyone to apply.
The graph applies to both consumers who cannot afford private insurance and consumers who choose not to purchase private insurance.
The government cannot discriminate!

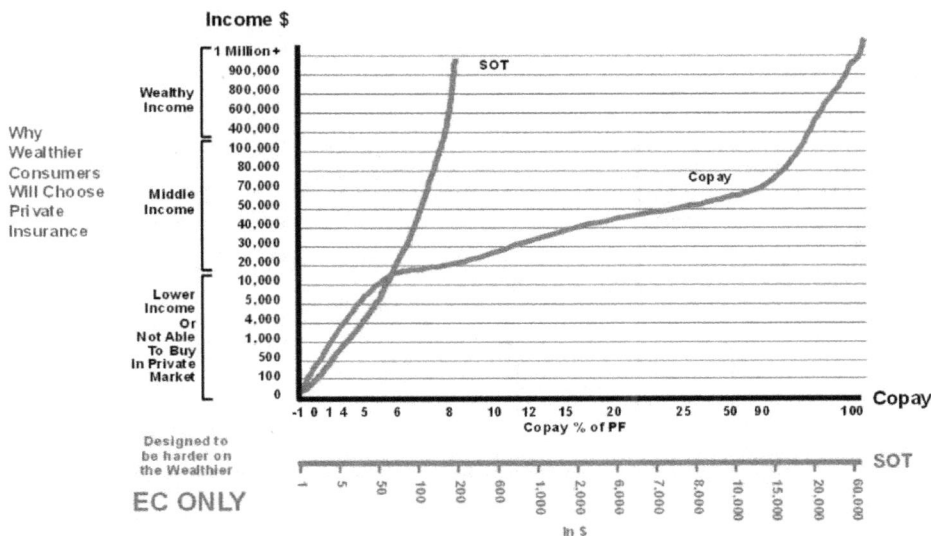

The graph below demonstrates why someone who could afford private insurance would not want the assigned plan. It would cause such a person to pay a higher co-pay and be required to go for more confirmatory second opinions than what a private plan would require for the same premium. The assigned plan is based solely on income, while the private insurance market is based on consumer choice.

On the other hand, it would offer very low co-pays and reasonable second opinion requirements for low income households. Just by the shape of the curves and their slopes the entire system can be implemented and maintained easily.

The reader is reminded to recall that all of these graphs and cards apply exclusively to elective care and that the graphs are representations for illustrative purposes. The actual graph will be generated by actuarial calculations.

Assigned Plan

Behind the Scenes Actuary Calculated Graph. This is how simple it can be!
This graph is meant only to simulate the mechanism.

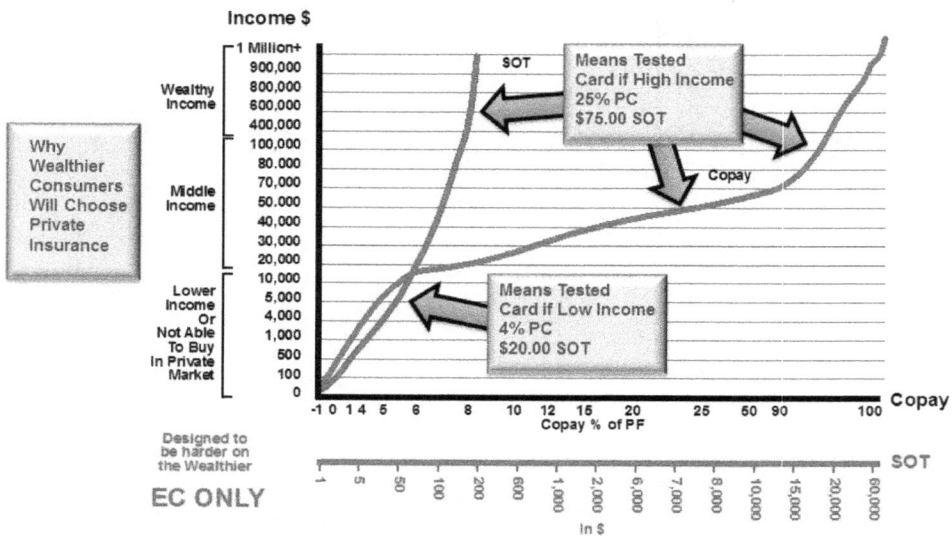

The government website to facilitate low income households in obtaining assigned insurance cards for elective care would look something like this:

Review Slide
How Does The Government
Apply a Universal Means Test?

Go to Hospital &/or Hospital Outreach
Clinic Intake/Reception or Web Site

Sum of All Sources of Income	Proof of Income	Zip	Sign Fraud Statement	Means PC	Means SOT
$____ $____ $____ Total $____	____ ____ ____ ____	____	"I affirm under penalty of the law..." Yes ____ No ____	____ ____ ____ ____	____ ____ ____ ____

Who Can Apply for Assigned Insurance?
Anyone or Everyone

Means tested income will likely produce higher PC & SOT
than private carriers for wealthier

This user-friendly website will be accessed by anyone and also used by the hospital intake desk when they provide consumers with a means tested assigned insurance card.

Both the government and private insurance plans compete, but in very different demographic markets where private insurance would not want to be and where government insurance has to be because the funding is so very different.

Reminder: the website that insurance companies provide, you may recall, looks very similar, but the underlying curves used to generate these user-friendly websites are very different.

Chapter 18: Specific issues and how they would be addressed within the IHPA of 2017

How does the system handle chronic illness?

- Diabetes
- Chronic heart problems
- Bipolar patients
- Thyroid patients
- Certain non-lethal tumor patients, etc.

By rewarding the patient directly for achieving certain goals. For example:

- Weight Loss
- Exercise
- Medication Compliance
- Accessing any form of preventative care or preventative testing
- Etc.

The plan acknowledges success with rewards programs similar to miles programs for credit cards.

The patients that improve their own state of health get immediate reduction in their co-pay and increase in their SOT.

How will the system handle huge hospital costs?

How can a normal patient afford to pay even his % co-pay (PC)

---

of a huge hospital bill generated by an elective stay?

- Even though hospitals are Providers, they compete on the basis of their day-stay rates.
- Consumers can shop and select the most cost effective hospital or surgicenter for elective procedures and workups.
- Most doctors work at several facilities.
- Furthermore, additional hospital cost controls remain in place.
- And most importantly, the patient will only be responsible for a small percentage (perhaps 20%) of the patient's percent co-pay (PC) identified on the patient's insurance card.

(e.g.: Hospital bill for elective admission is $10,000. Patient has a 10% co-pay, 10% of 10,000=$1,000. But hospital can only bill patients 20% of their PC (20% of $1,000=$200).

How does the system handle routine check-ups and preventative care?

This is obviously elective care and subject to PC and SOT. However these fees are usually below the common SOT. These services can be shopped and "good behavior" will provide rewards (via PC reduction) directly to the patient via the "Rewards Program."

How does the system handle fraud and abuse?

How does the plan control for excessive fees for UC or for providers stretching the definition of UC for things that are not really urgent?

The same way we handle fraud & abuse and price fixing now:

with severe penalties and investigation of red flags and alerts.

Also, if all the UC bills are going to the same place it will be much easier to identify the fraudulent behavior.

How does the plan handle cancer patients?

Very well! Cancer is usually life-threatening. Therefore, all patients with an established cancer diagnosis fall under the definition of UC. They are not required to pay their PC nor obligated to abide by their SOT.

However, the workup needed to arrive at the cancer diagnosis does come under the definition of elective care.

Cancer workup = Elective Care

Cancer treatment = Urgent or Catastrophic

Other Controversial Issues:

After appropriate laws are complied with, the specialty committees along with government will define which diagnoses are elective and which are not.

Robert Dennis, MD

Chapter 19: **Summation**

This concept is by no means fully packaged. It requires further input by other experts, and from all six players. The country's healthcare is vital to all of us. It should not be imposed upon us, but rather each of us needs to participate in the process and make it better. Inputs from all sectors and all participants are vital at this juncture so that the final outcome, with full appreciation for how painful change can be, will be the best it can be and far better than any other country's healthcare program.

There is a temptation to compare our country to others. This is simply not valid when it comes to healthcare. Just because other developed countries have universal healthcare does not mean you can extract that one piece of another society and transplant it here unless you look at all the other components of that society and adopt them as well.

We are a unique country and one size does not fit all. For example, other societies are not burdened with the same malpractice litigation concerns as are we. Therefore, if we adopt, for instance, Norway's health system we must also adopt their legal system. Actually, we can and should do better than has ever been done elsewhere rather than aim at mimicking another country's flawed plan. That is not good enough.

The U.S. can and will set the bar higher, by example, than other countries. The world will mimic us as it relates to quality, availability and access when we implement the IHPA of 2017.

SUMMARY

1. **When and if** this new paradigm, or parts of it, **ever become** part of a new guideline is of course pure conjecture.

2. But, with some tweaking and expansion it might reach 500 pages of simplicity which is better than 3000 pages of silly complication

Key Characteristics of The Informed Health Plan

- Easy to understand and implement

- **Enhances patient's choice** and the doctor/patient relationship

- Assumes that both **rich and poor are equally able to make informed healthcare decisions** (in the same way that we decide which TV, food, or appliance to purchase – **value vs. price (we are good at this)**

- Relies on **legitimate second opinions** instead of: rationing committees, government penalties, subsidies, referrals, authorizations, provider networks, deductibles and bureaucratic obstructions, etc.

Our Current Healthcare System Is Flawed

THE **INFORMED HEALTH PLAN**
FIXES IT

- Patients are disconnected from cost of care. Most are afraid to even ask the price, and others don't care because it is free to them or a third party pays.

- People do not have freedom to choose their healthcare providers based on quality and price. The scope of service is poorly defined, and there is limited competition among providers.

- Insurance coverage is inconsistent and there are too many opportunities for fraud.

    Reform is not a question, but a necessity.

- The **Informed Health Plan** uses technology to create transparency, clarity, and competition to empower the patient.

- If people can navigate the maze of purchasing a house, a car, or a refrigerator when given the pertinent facts, people **CAN** purchase healthcare when given the pertinent facts.

- Consumers **CAN** shop for healthcare and "vote with their feet" by accessing a searchable internet database for elective care with clearly defined prices posted by all providers.

- We **CAN** remove bureaucracy and delays instead of creating more bureaucracy and delays.

- We already pay for the uninsured through an ad hoc system that charges $4 for an Aspirin. We **CAN** efficiently provide quality care for the uninsured.

- We **CAN** reduce fraud, abuse, and unnecessary procedures.

- We **CAN** significantly reduce costs.

SUMMATION OF THE BENEFITS OF THE INFORMED DECISION HEALTHCARE PLAN

1. **Re-connect** people with their money.

2. Allow the **free market** to bring down prices.

3. Re-install meaningful **competition** among all providers.

4. Promote a means for people to **shop value** for healthcare.

5. **Empower consumers.**

6. Allow people to have **freedom of choice**.

7. Allow **people to decide** what they need and how much they want to pay.

8. Allow people to decide what **quality of life** means to them.

9. **Reduce fraud and abuse** in the system.

10. Provide a mechanism for real **transparency**.

11. Require something from all participants.

12. Access to all, but not completely free to anyone.

13. Define the terms "Urgent Care", "Catastrophic Care" as differentiated from "Elective Care."

14. Preserve programs that work

    - Such as **preventative programs**.

    - **Healthcare savings plan**

15. Stop hidden outrageous fees.

16. Stop different fees for different payors.

CHANGE YES, BUT CHANGE FOR THE BETTER!

Chapter 20: Stakeholder Advantages and Disadvantages

There are advantages and disadvantages produced for each stakeholder as a result of the various individual elements of the Informed Health Plan.

Government - Advantages

1. Provide access to all.
2. Reduce medical costs along with national debt.
3. Maintain control without micro-managing but rather by definitions.

Insurance Companies – Advantages

1. Increase profits.
2. Provide better product.
3. Improved image.
4. Be viewed as part of the solution.
5. Provide freedom of choice.
6. Provide more transparency.

Hospitals and Surgicenters – Advantages

1. Will receive 100% of their posted fees.
2. Simplified billing and prompt payment.
3. No more contracting for individual insurance companies for different pricing.

4. Will have increased revenue from new profit center. The hospital-run outreach clinics will serve the uninsured and bill the uninsured fund, while collecting only the means-tested fee from the patient.

Attorneys – Advantages

1. Improve their image by self-policing and being more accountable.
2. Enjoy reliable incomes with less stress.
3. Lower their investment in fruitless litigation (by accepting more winning suits).
4. Have an excuse to potential clients as to why they will not accept cases.
5. Enjoy lower healthcare premiums for their own staff.

Providers – Advantages

1. Increase hourly income and decrease stress.
2. Post and be paid in full the fees that they set for themselves (every time, without reduction, or repricing, or network reductions).
3. Ability to adjust fees and to verify their qualifications and reviews annually on a government website.
4. Improve doctor/patient relationship by eliminating obstructive and costly bureaucratic and intrusive micro-management.
5. Increase patient volume and decrease malpractice exposure (by their willingness to promote voluntary and mandatory second opinions).

Patients – Advantages

1. Dramatically increase meaningful, knowledgeable information about their own medical conditions.
2. Empowered to make better, more informed decisions based on cost, quality, and medical need for all elective decisions (will have the tools to shop for insurance and providers).
3. Enjoy dramatically decreased medical costs and increased quality of care.
4. Have the ability to see any willing licensed provider, in any state.
5. Less paperwork and fewer delays and obstructions to care.

Disadvantages

Government – Disadvantages

1. Less intrusive control.
2. Less bureaucracy.
3. Fewer patronage jobs.
4. More transparency.

Insurance companies – Disadvantages

1. Lose immunity to malpractice litigation.
2. Lose micro-management control and be removed as a 3rd party in the exam room.
3. Contribute a percentage of the premium to the uninsured pool.

4. Contribute a percentage of the premium to the urgent and catastrophic pool.

5. Compete with each other on only two parameters.

Hospitals and Surgicenters – Disadvantages

1. Compete with each other on price and quality directly to the consumer and physician.

2. Establish simplified fee structure with a few exceptions:
   a. Day rate for a given procedure
   b. Day rate for complex procedures
   c. Day rate for extended stay

3. Post all fees on government website. Distribute fee schedules to all doctors' offices, both doctors on staff and local doctors not on staff.

4. Triage and redirect in the ER
   a. Patients with catastrophic conditions for treatment or admission, OR
   b. All other patients (for elective care) to the outreach clinics or to the patient's private doctor.

5. All hospitals are required to establish specialty specific outreach clinics.

Attorneys – Disadvantages

1. Increased malpractice premiums.

2. Reduction in volume of malpractice cases.

3. Reduction in size of settlements.

Providers – Disadvantages

1. Compete on price, qualifications, reputation, and bedside manner.
2. Be subject to peer review scrutiny via frequent second opinions.
3. Incur the potential loss of a patient to the voluntary or mandatory second opinion doctor.

Patients – Disadvantages

1. Will need to reset their approach by taking the responsibility to shop, think and be accountable for medical decisions. (In other words, get more involved and be a better consumer.)
2. Pay the designated co-pay at the time of service for **all** care except urgent/catastrophic care which requires no co-pay.
3. Make time to obtain the voluntary or mandatory specialty-specific second opinion for elective care only.
4. Self-ration perceived demands which now must be substituted by their personal, better-informed medical need determinants.

Executive Summary

Informed Health Plan Act of 2017

Major points only – Please see detailed plan.
www.InformedHealthPlan.com

A. Providers: Post all fees and qualifications
B. Health Insurance Companies:

1. Contribute to two pools:
   a. Uninsured pool
   b. Catastrophic pool
2. Pay providers posted fees
3. Sell plans that vary only by co-pay amounts and the threshold amounts required for mandatory second opinions
4. Encourage savings plans
5. Portable state-to-state plans
6. No pre-existing illness clauses
7. No more restrictive provider networks

C. Attorneys:
   1. Tort Reform
      a. Caps for pain and suffering
      b. Police themselves via a "practical" new definition of frivolous suit, with reasonable penalties if all 3 criteria are met

D. Patients (Below age 65):
   1. Shop price and quality
   2. Pay something for each piece of healthcare no matter how little
   3. Have a "Living Will"
   4. Second opinions for non-urgent care over a "patient's selected" threshold amount

E. Hospitals:
   1. Post all fees and expect to compete on price and quality.
   2. Establish and run outreach clinics funded via a fund called "Uninsured Fund." See detailed plan.

F. Government:
   1. Define terms (urgent, non-urgent, and catastrophic

care) and regulate system as provided by this new legislation and not beyond

2. Leave Medicare ALONE!

3. Proportionally fund two pools of funds along with substantial contributions from insurance companies and state government, etc.

   a. Uninsured pool

   b. Catastrophic pool

4. Expand COBRA and health savings plans

5. Transparency for all health related revenue sources

The Informed Health Plan Act of 2017

Remember our

"Buy One, Send One Free" Offer

Don't Delay!

With your purchase of this book, follow the instructions below and we will send a copy of The Informed Health Plan Act of 2017 to your legislator – at no cost to you.

Please also visit our website for updates and additional information, including videos from author Dr. Robert Dennis and various social media links.

To send a copy of The Informed Health Plan Act of 2017, please visit:

www.InformedHealthPlan.com

Click on "Send A Free Copy To My Legislator" link in the top right corner.

Add your first name and ZIP Code and we will send a free copy to your legislator.

---

www.ingramcontent.com/pod-product-compliance
Lightning Source LLC
Chambersburg PA
CBHW051413200326
41520CB00023B/7214